Women's Midlife Anim-Morphosis

Unlock your Inner Power and be Present to Your Life

Lea Ausch Alteras Ph.D.

Author of Three Generations of Jewish Women: Holocaust
Survivors, Their Daughters, and Granddaughters

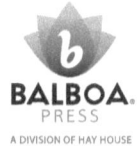

BALBOA.
PRESS

A DIVISION OF HAY HOUSE

Balboa Press books may be ordered through booksellers or by contacting:

Balboa Press
A Division of Hay House
1663 Liberty Drive
Bloomington, IN 47403
www.balboapress.com
1 (877) 407-4847

Because of the dynamic nature of the Internet, any web addresses or links contained in this book may have changed since publication and may no longer be valid. The views expressed in this work are solely those of the author and do not necessarily reflect the views of the publisher, and the publisher hereby disclaims any responsibility for them.

The author of this book does not dispense medical advice or prescribe the use of any technique as a form of treatment for physical, emotional, or medical problems without the advice of a physician, either directly or indirectly. The intent of the author is only to offer information of a general nature to help you in your quest for emotional and spiritual well-being. In the event you use any of the information in this book for yourself, which is your constitutional right, the author and the publisher assume no responsibility for your actions.

Any people depicted in stock imagery provided by Thinkstock are models, and such images are being used for illustrative purposes only. Certain stock imagery © Thinkstock.

Print information available on the last page.

ISBN: 978-1-5043-5539-1 (sc)
ISBN: 978-1-5043-5541-4 (hc)
ISBN: 978-1-5043-5540-7 (e)

Library of Congress Control Number: 2016906171

Balboa Press rev. date: 08/11/2016

Contents

I wish to dedicate this book to my grandchildren: Lauren, Samantha, Jack, Estella, Mila, and Lucy

Acknowledgements

I am filled with a sense of gratitude as I reflect upon the support and encouragement my family and friends provided me with throughout the years it took to write this book.

First and foremost, to my daughter Debbie: thanks for your creativity, advice, and unconditional support that gave me the strength to go on. Watching you develop into the generous and hard-working woman that you are today makes me proud to be your mother.

To my husband Isaac: thank you for being a source of comfort throughout the sometimes grueling process of writing and research. Your own accomplishments spurred my own pursuits.

To my son Robert: thank you for being my role-model. Watching your continuous growth as a thinker and your thirst for knowledge and wisdom paved the way toward my own love of learning.

To my six grandchildren: thank you for being the loving, sweet souls that you are and for reminding me what truly matters in life. Watching you grow, gave me the motivation to write this book and to impart to you knowledge on matters facing today's women.

To my co-workers, friends, and all the women I interviewed: thank you for the advice and insights that you provided, which helped me understand more clearly the anxieties that most of us women experience at this juncture of our lives (i.e., middle age).

Introduction

"Age is an issue of mind over matter. If you don't mind it, it does not matter."

Mark Twain

My big awakening came at my sixtieth birthday. Throughout my adult life I have exited each year of my lifecycle with ease and joy, until my surprise sixtieth birthday party when a sense of confusion and sadness overwhelmed me. Suddenly, I realized that old age is knocking at my door, bringing social security benefits, half-priced movie tickets, and retirement just around the corner. I felt that this birthday was my tipping point between youth and age, moving me from a younger generation to a senior one. I could no longer deny the fact that I was aging, no matter how hard I tried to stay young.

As I approached my sixties, I realized that many of my conversations with friends and women my age focused on "confusing moments" about topics related to our aging process: our appearance, identity, values, roles, priorities, relationships, finances, work, hormonal changes, and physical and mental wellbeing. Certainly, as I advanced in age I expected changes within my body and mind, but I found that these changes caused me unnecessary anxiety, stress, and confusion because of the wrath that society directs at aging woman.

Middle-aged women are bombarded with the message that life is over after fifty. At fifty, women are expected to lack vitality, curiosity, passion, excitement, interests and zest for life. It's a time of rapid mental and physical decline. Repeatedly I heard the message that middle-age is a time for retirement and leisure. My changing body, combined with the message that society was directing at me, forced me to question my role in society and my trajectory moving forward. I was guilty of absorbing the ageism in our culture, which was depressing me. The thought of living the next twenty years of my life in anticipation and preparation for death seemed hopeless and futile. Before I could begin my journey toward embracing a healthy concept of age and aging, I had to make peace with the warped attitudes that I had unconsciously internalized throughout my sixty years of living.

My blood would boil every time a young man would call me "Ma'am" or give me his seat on the subway. Being viewed as "elderly" was difficult for me to accept. But slowly, I started discovering that a healthy part of aging is to accept all the attendant experiences, embracing both the thirty-five-year-old who still lives inside of me and the sixty-year-old body that I inhabit. I felt that life had more in store for me, and I was on a mission to find out what that was. Questions swarmed in my head: Who am I? What has happened to my face, body, and mind? I realized that much of my confusion originated from the messages that I had internalized as a child. In the traditional family and community I grew up in, a strong emphasis was placed on my exterior looks with little regard for my interior wellbeing, i.e. my inner-self. It took me many years to integrate my inner and outer worlds, making them both integral parts of my personality.

At sixty I find myself at a crossroad. A new stage of life is unfolding where most of my past roles are coming to an end. I am confused and anxious on the one hand, yet extremely excited to discover the new me. Learning new things at any age in life is both exciting and frightening. I realized that I needed to rethink and revise the ageist messages that I was regularly inundated with on billboards, commercials, musical lyrics, magazines and T.V. shows. I searched among the aisles of countless bookstores and book providers, and I was unable to find a comprehensive guide or manual to combat the negative perceptions associated with aging women. Our society's assumption is that "youth is best" or at least "younger is better." As a result, I determined that I no longer want to be identified by my chronological age. Who wants to view themselves as undesirable, void of fertility, sexuality and productivity? I realized that the negative myths associated with age were at the root of my confusion. This revelation forced me to challenge society's outdated views and its misconceptions about myself and other women in their middle-life, and it jolted me to gain some knowledge and understanding of my own aging process.

I constantly reminded myself that although the concept of middle-age seems like a universal truth, it is a fabricated creation. There is little consensus by the mass media and advertising companies regarding when middle-age begins, how long it lasts, or when it ends. Both the media and the advertising world use this so-called "middle-age" for marketing purposes. The message that they promote is clear: "Once you use our recommended products, services, medical procedures or youth-enhancing drugs, you can slow down or stop your aging process." These days, middle-age onscreen and in magazines looks thinner, smoother, sexier, wealthier, and happier than ever. These perpetually improved middle-aged women tone their bodies at daily workouts, freeze their faces, lunch at expensive restaurants and dress more like teenagers. But this imagined middle-age is just that: "imagined." In reality middle-age is brimming with opportunities and disappointments that include the size six and the size eighteen, the enthusiastic entrepreneur and the anxious laid-off worker, the single mother and the retired grandmother. These contradictory images of aging deepened my confusions about my own aging process and led me to feelings of ambiguity about what is appropriate at my age. In order to continue along the path of self-discovery, my goal became to debunk the old myopic messages regarding middle-age that I had internalized and bring some clarity into my life and the lives of my generation of women, the "baby boomers."

I must admit that it's hard to grow old in a culture devoted to staying young. I began my exploration with many questions. How do I gain understanding of what it means to be "not young"? How do I challenge the negative images directed at aging women? How do I bring to light the strength and courage that my generation of women possess? These are but a few of the questions that began to overwhelm me and needed my immediate attention. At that moment, I knew that writing this book would help me find the answers to my questions as well as help other middle-aged women facing similar questions. Like many women, I was once filled with fear – fear that limited my options. I realized that my waiting, wishing and blaming kept me a hostage for many years. I needed to be proactive and take charge of my life. I needed to break out of my fear zone and rewrite my inner narrative. Most importantly, I needed to realize that in some ways I had learned to be afraid by internalizing false assumptions and attitudes about age.

Despite the media's obsession with youth, the psychologists Carl Jung (1968) and Erik Erikson (1967) both maintain that middle-age propels us toward our greatest achievements. Carl Jung claims that a "human being would certainly not grow to be seventy or eighty years old if this longevity had no meaning... The afternoon of life must have significance of its own and cannot be merely a pitiful appendage of life's morning." (p. 42) He emphasizes the fact that the second part of our lives is to sustain our culture and provide wisdom to the next generation. It's also a time for changes, growth, and discoveries. It's a time to re-examine our lives, roles, and position in our society. I call this self-reevaluation and transformation "anim-morphosis," and for it to be successful we need the wisdom that we acquired throughout our lives. Middle-aged baby boomers, myself included, have something previous generations did not have, and that is more time due to longer life spans. Those of us in the middle have decades to recoup losses and change directions. Aging is not our enemy, as many of us perceive it, but rather a time to shed old identities and embrace new ones. It's a time when we can let go of past grievances, make peace with ourselves, get rid of old baggage, explore new options, and move forward with a lighter load.

We have at our disposal hundreds of books written on the subject of middle-age, but there is no comprehensive book that directly addresses its onset, progression and duration. Since more and more women are working through this long turbulent period with little information about its progression, I took it upon myself to write this book to help myself and other women struggling through the process of aging. My mission in writing this book is to acquire a deeper understanding of the concept called "middle-age." When does it start? When does it end? How long does it last? If we don't talk about it honestly, then how and where do we learn about it? If society's attitude is that this is an age of decline and there is nothing positive about it, then how can we face it and live through it? As I started searching through the literature, I was astonished to find the way middle-age was defined as an "exact age" without clear explanations as to the different sub-stages during this long period. Most theories of development concentrate on defining the earlier stages of our lifecycles while ignoring the later stages of adult life. It's time to understand and expand our knowledge of this long lifecycle and broaden our views of its different sub-stages.

The cultural assumption is that once we hit the age of twenty-something and we become young adults there are few changes to come. This false assumption creates a void in the study of adult development. With no map to guide me, I decided to fill in all the missing pieces and explore specific concerns that I and other middle-aged women face. I began by making a clear distinction between the different sub-stages of middle-age: early middle-age (late forties to early fifties), mid-middle-age (late fifties to early sixties) and late middle-age (late sixties to mid-seventies). Just as in our adolescence, middle-age is beset by changes of enormous magnitude. Consciously or unconsciously, we have to acknowledge that our lives as we have known them no longer exist. We are faced with many life changes including divorce, empty nest, loss of a job that defined us for many years, changes in our appearance, bulges around our waists, wrinkles, thinning hair, altering health, and so on. But the argument that I present in this book is that we can compensate for many of these changes by using our inner power that lies dormant, just waiting to be awakened. Middle-age is giving us an opportunity to do things differently and learn to let go of who we are in order to become who we want to be.

I hope that as you read through the chapters of this book you will find helpful information, suggestions, exercises, and research on issues concerning your life. This book serves multiple functions depending on your individual needs. Some of you will use this book as a guide to improve your physical and/or emotional wellbeing, while others may use this book to clarify one specific area of confusion. Regardless, this book will help you gain insight, knowledge, self-awareness and important guidance for self-discovery as you advance through the middle and later years of your life. This book embraces a "do it yourself approach," i.e., self-coaching, for reshaping both your inner and outer life. Since we are all unique individuals, each of us needs to take an individualistic approach to our own discoveries of life at middle-age and beyond. We are all born with the power of self-discovery. We just need some guidance on how to tap into it and create a unique personalized life-plan. Throughout the book, I refer to this self-journey as "anim-morphosis," which is a term that means self-change.

This book offers a holistic approach to wellness and health. A holistic approach to health emphasizes all parts of our existence: psychological, physical, social, environmental, and spiritual. When we think of our bodies, minds, hair, skin, they all belong to the same unit. For example, healthy skin begins with a healthy mind, healthy heart, healthy liver and so on. What this means is that we need to focus on our mental health, nutrition, exercise, stress relief, and eliminate all toxicities from our lives in order for our skin to radiate. Having a positive mind-set would help us make healthy choices about nutrition, exercise, skincare, and social life. We would be able to fully concentrate on how our bodies feel and what we truly need to look and feel healthy.

This book not only explores mid-adulthood in women's lives but also explores the way in which the extended period of health and activity achieved by modern science has expanded the contributions that women make during middle life. Middle adulthood is a period in which accumulated experience is combined with health and energy. Continued health during mid-life offers us choices that were not available to previous generations. These choices reflect the ongoing ways in which women shape and reshape their lives, intuitively seeking balance, peace, and fulfillment. With the expanded horizon that lies before us, we have every reason to be grateful. Instead of complaining about age, we ought to enjoy the extra time, especially since the added years haven't been tacked on to the end of our lives but are ours to enjoy in the middle. Happily, it is middle-age that has lengthened so that most peoples' fifties and sixties are a continuum of high energy living. Today in our society there is what we call the "boomer surplus," a major increase in the demographic landscape for people between fifty and seventy-five. The 2014 U.S. Census figures offers compelling data on this population increase, an increase that results both from larger numbers of people in the boomer cohort, including my generation (born between 1945 to 1950), and from greater life expectancy due to scientific and medical advances.

Some of us boomers are already reaping the benefits of this new knowledge. We believe that age is irrelevant, myself included. What is relevant is function and ability. We posses an innate desire to stay healthy, fit, and mentally alert because we know that our lives will be fuller, longer and filled with greater opportunity. This is the generation that has said "yes" to anti-aging medicine and decided that it has better things to do than sit around and get old. My generation of baby boomers has introduced the "fitness movement," which I hope will be recorded in history as being the forerunner to anti-aging medicine. We have made the commitment to keeping active for as long as possible. However, with this book, I intend to enlighten middle-age women who have not participated nor benefitted from this new anti-aging medicine. We need to throw away the old messages about aging and re-educate ourselves on the most up-to-date theories of how and why we age.

This extra time, as well as some of my generation's changing attitudes towards life and health, could be used to our advantage and create compensatory gains to offset the losses of aging. For example, our vision, our skin elasticity, and our bone density will inevitably diminish, but we can increase our physical strength, our stamina, speed up our metabolism, improve our eating habits, pay attention to our appearance, boost our self-confidence and self-acceptance, and revamp our image of ourselves. The image that we should embrace is that we are growing stronger, more competent and happier, not just older. If such awareness is not achieved, women are susceptible to having a mid-life crisis, which is nothing more than panicking over one's inability to control the variables later in life.

Every day we are faced with two distinct choices: to do something different and grow or to resist change because we are fueled by fear. Embracing growth and allowing for "anim-morphosis" are the keys to staying young. Growth is experienced through curiosity, discovery, challenge, commitment, and adversity. Letting go and embracing change will inevitably move us from the tyranny of "I ought to" to " I choose to." We need to arm ourselves against an undertow that continues to regard age as the decline of body, mind, and spirit. Women as early as forty feel differently about themselves, their bodies, their roles, and their places in society. These feelings are reinforced by the negative image of age rampant in our society, and they create in us a sense of confusion and at times anger. Our concern with how we look may be superficial, but it's natural. We should not feel ashamed about obsessing over appearance occasionally, since this is a time in our lives when our youthful looks are fading. Let's not brush it under the rug as something superficial that will pass. Our changing bodies, our wrinkles, our menopause, and the end of our fertile years are realities that we need to accept if we are to enjoy our middle adulthood and beyond. This book provides a blueprint that will help you progress through mid-life with choices and visions. Many women, myself included, have lost their way and are eager to find a satisfactory path as they age. This book is unique, because it provides a comprehensive guide, including exercises, suggestions and valuable research on important topics that most middle-age women need at this juncture in their lives. It is anchored on the premise that self-confidence, physical stamina, mental stamina, and self-grooming have value at any age and that they are interconnected. This simply means that we have to pay attention to all aspects of ourselves if we are to enjoy our full potential as we progress through middle-age and beyond.

This book's chapters focus on different aspects of women's lives, such as self-esteem, nutrition, exercise, mental endurance, skincare, clothing, de-cluttering, stress management, goal attainment, and many more. Even though each chapter deals with a specific topic, they are all interconnected. The unifying concept is the integration of our inner and outer lives. Our inner lives entail self-awareness, self-acceptance, self-esteem, respect, self-discovery and self-worth, while our outer lives deal with relationships to people, our community, our environment, nutrition, exercise, hygiene, aesthetics, and appearance. The process of growth moves in both directions, from inner growth to outer growth and vice-versa. This mind-body approach emphasizes a balance between our inner selves, the way we feel about ourselves, and our outer selves, the way we are perceived by others.

Chapter One deals with stages of development. Since at every stage in our lifecycle we experience specific crises, it is important for us to gain awareness of what those crises are and learn ways to resolve them. If we do not make the transitions from stage to stage successfully, we will carry remnants of those crisis for the rest of our lives and diminish our quality of life.

Chapter Two deals with our body-mind interconnection. Understanding that our thoughts, beliefs, feelings and emotions fuel every cell in our body and that nothing holds more power over our bodies than our minds is the major focus of this chapter. These interconnections are at the roots of our existence.

Chapter Three deals with "the self" and addresses the question of who we are. It provides us with different methods of mending our self-esteem, which is key to staying young and healthy. A healthy mind creates a healthy body, and a health body and mind create a healthy life. For example, I examine the connection between our inner voices and low self-esteem. Learning how to disarm our inner critical voice that discourages us from growth and change is crucial to freeing ourselves and raising our self-esteem. Our inner voice carries the feelings we were unable to express as a child. It carries our anger, shame, fear, excitement, joy and love. Somehow we have learned as children to ignore or deny those feelings. Part of this process explores how to make accurate self-assessments of our strengths and weaknesses, as well as identify our irrational thinking. Challenging and changing our thinking is one of the most powerful ways of undoing old negative programming and freeing ourselves to live mindfully instead of mindlessly. I call this process "inner anim-morphosis," or inner self-change.

Chapter Four focuses on our brain power. How do we keep our brains agile and strong throughout our lifecycle? And how do we increase our brain stamina at this point in our lives? This chapter provides the reader with the necessary tools and guidance to achieve this goal by providing evidence that our brain plasticity can be maintained throughout our lifespan. In this chapter, I make the argument that an active brain and body keep us alert and healthy throughout our lives.

Chapter Five deals with enhancing our physical stamina. Maintaining our stamina through physical exercises and active living encourages our vitality and keeps our mental and physical strength alive. The theme of this chapter is captured by a quote from the great feminist writer Adrienne Rich: "I know of no woman for whom the body is not a fundamental problem." Having internalized our bodies as a problem is at the heart of women's health; changing our perceptions of our bodies is at the heart of our healing process. The secret to thriving is the knowledge that we are never simply victims of our bodies, and we have within us the ability to heal from anything and go on to live joy-filled lives.

Chapter Six examines the importance that nutrition plays in our health and well-being. The big question addressed throughout this chapter is "How do we adjust our eating habits, lifestyle, activity level, and attitudes to keep a strong and healthy body and mind in middle-age?" My main argument is that there is no such thing as a diet. All diets fail because they work on a self-deprivation principle. We need to change our mind-set from self-deprivation to self-fulfillment by developing an individualized eating plan "fit for life." We need to be able to distinguish between healthy foods and unhealthy foods; between foods that deplete us from energy and those that give us energy; between foods that make us anxious as opposed to foods that make us calm. Once we acquire this knowledge, we can develop our own individualized eating plan.

Beginning the second part of the book, Chapter Seven focuses on our outer appearance, which depends on the strength of our inner beauty. We cannot look good on the outside if we neglect our inside. If we feel depressed, our faces will look tired, and our bodies will be void of energy and vitality. But if we eat nutritious food, exercise, keep our minds active, sleep well, and reduce our stress level, our skin glows and our hair shines. Our skin, hair, nails and teeth have a dynamic interaction with the health of the rest of our body. A frail body equates to frail skin, and a healthy body and mind equates to glowing skin and hair.

Chapter Eight deals with our psychology of dressing. There is no stronger evidence of the interconnection between our minds and bodies than our psychology of dressing, which means that the way we dress is the way we feel. Our language of fashion expresses the way we feel about ourselves and the way we want to be perceived by those around us. When we shop, we consider our size, lifestyle, age, and environment. We either work to incorporate all these aspects into our dressing style or we work against them. Our closets reflect this simple reality.

Chapter Nine focuses on methods to eliminate all the toxicities that we have accumulated throughout our lives. Examining what works and what does not, what's missing and what needs to be eliminated, will help us move on with a lighter load. We need to familiarize ourselves with both our inner and outer toxicities, such as fear, guilt, control, shame, toxic relationships, a toxic work environment, poor time management, financial chaos, and so on.

Chapter Ten addresses the importance of setting goals and putting them into action. Just having a goal, envisioning a change, or even creating a plan doesn't get us there. Middle-age is our time to take charge of our lives by developing specific action plans, following them through, and getting results. We are wiser about our likes and dislikes, our strengths and weaknesses, as well as our self-sabotaging thoughts and behaviors. So changing the things that don't work well in our lives is up to us.

This book is not about how you ought to grow older, but rather a candid report on what it's really like to age. It details some new ways of thinking about and dealing with age through becoming an active participant in the process. I believe that life provides us with two doors: one door leads to resistance and the other door leads to growth. If you feel ready to walk through the second, more challenging door, walk with me and remember that "openness" is the key that unlocks it.

The mere fact that you're holding this book means that you're interested in "anim-morphosis." However, before you begin your journey, ask yourself: What is my current concept of getting older? What are my feelings about embarking on this journey? Do I think people are capable of real change? Do I think that I am capable of change? Be honest about your answers. Study them and you'll prepare your mind to be open to the ideas that this book presents.

My experience will not be your experience. Each one of us is unique and we experience mid-life in different ways. For example, some of us are immersed in lengthy careers while others experience major changes and embark upon new ventures. Some of us notice the subtle and not-so-subtle effects of aging on our bodies and minds, while others are in the best shape of their lives. Some of us may experience a crisis at midlife, while others may simply notice small changes in the way they feel about their lives or how they relate to others around them. One thing is certain: none of us will remain untouched at this point in our lives.

Learning to grow smarter and stronger each day as we navigate through our youth-obsessed society is what this book is all about. We need creativity, curiosity, playfulness, flexibility, and a strong willingness to venture into the unknown territories of age in order to master this period in our lives. I hope this book can offer assistance as you confront some of these challenges. My purpose in writing this book is to bring awareness and to provide strategies and exercises which could be tailored to fit your individual needs and lifestyle. I look at aging as an opportunity for greater love, wisdom, freedom, creativity, joy, and increased mental and physical capacity. This book is designed to be used as a manual for renewal with practical recommendations and practices at the conclusion of each chapter.

You are about to embark upon an adventure that will reward you for the rest of your life. You are going to learn new ways to break the bonds that have been holding you back. If you find yourself in a situation where you seem to be going nowhere, this book is for you. If you are disgusted with mediocrity, disappointed by past results, and not content to just drift through life, these pages offer you an alternative. If you make yourself open and receptive to new concepts, values, and beliefs, you will discover how you can systematically reorganize your thoughts to awaken "the new you." Once you master these principles, you will have more freedom, love, and self-confidence than you ever thought possible.

The great psychologist Carl Rogers (1961) concluded that nothing is more rewarding than unleashing your fullest potential and leading a creative, purposeful life. It makes no difference who you are, what you do or what your life situation is. You can achieve self-renewal, i.e. anim-morphosis, and the approach is not nearly as complicated as you might think!

It took me five years to write this book, not because of lack of motivation, but rather because that was how long it took me to see through my own deceptions, lies, excuses and pain. My rational being understood that unless I got to the underlying reason of why I was struggling, I couldn't move forward. As I began, I started seeing things differently and understood that my misguided perceptions were victimizing my life. Life did not victimize me, but rather how I interpreted, thought and reacted to my life became the reasons I was stuck.

I realized that most of my common types of degeneration were the result of my lifestyle choices, the results of how I treated myself, including my brain and body. I started believing in anti-aging possibilities, and I incorporated lifestyle changes and a proactive approach to my life. I kept my brain agile with daily activities, my body fit with daily exercises and healthy nutrition, my stress under control, my self-image positive, and I cleaned out all my mental clutter and toxicities. Once I accomplished these changes, I was able to move on with ease and clarity. Even though I have internalized many negative messages throughout my childhood years, the only thing that counts today are the present experiences which are within my reach.

Your Current Notions of Age

"One day I said to myself: I am forty. By the time I recovered from the shock of that discovery, I had reached fifty."

Simone de Beauvoir

Exercise I

Reflect upon your current notion of age by answering these questions:

When was the first time you noticed your appearance was changing?

What did you think at that moment?

Do you look in the mirror often?

What do you say to yourself about what you see?

Do you spend a long time getting ready to go out?

What words do you use to define beauty?

How does the culture of beauty impact you?

Do you feel competitive with other women your age or younger?

Do you like spending time with women your age or younger?

How do you feel when you are surrounded by women your age or older?

Do you have moments when you feel or think "I'm no longer young?"

Do you shy away from taking pictures?

What is your reaction when you see others looking at you?

Are you disappointed if people don't notice you?

Do you believe how you age is largely out of your control?

These simple questions zero in on how you perceive "age" and highlight some of the negative perceptions that you might have developed about aging which block your path to achieving your ideal experiences in life. If you believe that aging steals your youth, slows you down, hinders you from many activities, or that aging is completely out of your control, then each additional year in your life might cause you unnecessary stress. As you read through this book, you will develop an understanding of the difference between which aspects of aging you do have control over and which aspects you do not, which you can change and which you cannot, and how to develop a specific plan of action to deal with those things which you can change. I challenge you to discard any reservations you might have regarding aging and to take a more active role in your self-management.

The Price of Re-Inventing Your Life

Exercise II

Answer the following three questions:

Are you willing to do something active to change your life in addition to reading this book?

Do you believe that you could achieve positive changes in your life?

Do you want changes in your life?

Your answers can only be from a list of three possibilities:

Yes, I will do all the assignments.

No, I won't do them.

I haven't made up my mind yet.

If you answered yes, then you are on your way to embarking on a life-changing journey. If you answered no, it's important to examine the reasons you don't want to participate. For example, you might be overwhelmed by your negative self-talk with comments such as "I'm not convinced that the exercises will make a difference in my life," "I'm not ready to start now, but I might do them at a later date," "I'm afraid I'm not smart enough to do a good job," "I want to read the whole book and see if things make sense to me," or "I think these exercises are a waste of my time." Remember that the self-help exercises will be crucial to your success. So don't fight them, embrace them.

> "Life is like riding a bicycle to keep your balance: you must keep moving."

> Albert Einstein

Part I

CHAPTER I

Your Developmental Stages: Moving from Ignorance toward Wisdom

"The life which is unexamined is not worth living."

Plato

Since a big part of this book concentrates on our lifecycle, it is important that we understand our progression from birth through our entire life span. Understanding the origins of our self-esteem, becoming self-aware, having self-respect, and developing self-acceptance are all part of our growth toward adulthood. Last century, many psychologists labeled adolescence an important stage of development, a stage that creates a bridge between our childhood years and young adulthood. In the twenty-first century, another phase of life seems to be emerging as similarly significant, capturing our interest and expanding our understanding of human potential and development. Middle-age, which starts in our late forties and expands into our mid-seventies, creates a bridge between our early and late adulthood years. The people in this age range are redefining our views of human development. This is the age group that most developmental theories have neglected to study closely, and this book concentrates exclusively on it.

The willingness to move through each stage of our lives is equivalent to the willingness to live fully. Growth demands a temporary surrender of security. It may mean giving up a familiar but limiting pattern, which might feel uncomfortable at times. But the reward

3

will come later. As Dostoevsky said, "Taking a new step, uttering a new word is what people fear most" (Dostoevsky 1886, 96). The courage to move forward and take new steps allows us to let go of each stage by resolving our crises and enter a new stage of life with the potential for finding fresh ideas and richer life experiences.

The stages of development were studied extensively by three developmental psychologists, Erik Erikson (1963), Jean Piaget (1967) and Vygotsky (1978). While they all took different approaches, they all agreed that development is a continuous process of progress through stages, and each stage needs to be mastered successfully in order to move on to the next. Piaget looked upon development as an individual process first occurring within the child, while Vygotsky argued that development is a social process that occurs during social interaction with a person with a higher level of knowledge. He called this interaction "the zone of proximal development." Vygotsky claimed that "What the child can accomplish today with help, she can do alone tomorrow," which means that learning takes place through social interaction. Then, as learning becomes the child's own knowledge, the child internalizes it.

In his book *Childhood and Society* (1967), Erikson identified eight stages of development. He argued that each stage is characterized by a specific crisis that we need to resolve in order to move on to our next stage successfully. Every stage in our lifecycle has a beginning, a middle, and an end. At the beginning we start with baby steps similar to the ones we took in infancy. As we move on, we are faced with crises and challenges that strengthen our resolve as we learn to navigate our quest for self-fulfillment and wellness.

If we don't overcome our crises at the specific ages when they occur, we will carry the remnants of them into the next stage of our lifecycle, or all our lives, limiting our chances of achieving our fullest potentials (Rogers, 1961). I prefer to call these life crises "turning points" in our lives because they allow us to reflect and reexamine our life's purpose before moving on to our next stage of development.

Erikson (1967) recognized what emerges from the resolution of a crisis, or a turning point, at different stages of our lifecycle: trust, attachment, nurturance, and security during infancy; autonomy and will during early childhood; purpose, creativity, and freedom during play age; industry, competence, and cooperation during school age; identity, commitment, and exploration in adolescence; career, connections, and love in young adulthood; care, self-reflection, self-evaluation, transformation, growth, and compassion in middle adulthood; wisdom and acceptance in old age. Each of these strengths is prefigured at earlier stages, and each is reshaped to address the challenges of later stages.

Infancy

During infancy, we have to establish a trusting, safe, and nurturing relationship with parents and caregivers, but at the same time maintain enough distrust so that we are not left completely unprotected and vulnerable. This safe, nurturing, and trusting environment is a prerequisite for normal development and sets the foundation for the adult personality. If we are unable to develop trust, we will have issues around intimacy, trusting others, and holding on to relationships. We may even having a hard time trusting ourselves. The crisis that we develop at this stage is a sense of mistrust, and if not resolved later in life, it will hinder our existence. Our inability to experience safety in childhood could result in either seeking compulsive closeness or avoiding it for fear of getting rejected or hurt.

Our first relationships set the foundation for our next stage of development: autonomy versus shame and doubt. At this stage we develop our first sense of independence by walking, vocalizing, and exploring the environment—we can begin to do things on our own. But if this sense of autonomy is discouraged, restricted, or ridiculed we will develop a sense of shame and doubt that could haunt us for the rest of our lives.

By age three, we are figuring out how to relate to others, and we start learning what to do to get what we need. But if we grow up in a dysfunctional family where our needs have not been met or we have been ridiculed for having them, we may not learn how to have our needs fulfilled, thereby reinforcing our negative feelings of shame. Many of the negative messages we internalize and take ownership of as adults originate from early messages from significant adults. For example, our feelings of shame, fear, guilt, doubt, self-criticism, and the need for perfection originate in this stage of development. This is the stage that defines the people who won't try anything new for fear of failing or being ridiculed. They have no confidence in their ability, and they seem to deny their needs because they might have been ridiculed as children for having them.

Early Childhood

Early childhood is a period when our sense of initiative or sense of guilt develops. At this stage we comprehend that we are a person, an individual, and now we must discover what kind of person we will become. We identify intensely with our parents, who, most of the time, appear to us to be powerful and unreasonable. We have a surplus of energy that permits us to forget failure quickly and to approach new areas that seem desirable, even if dangerous. At this stage of development, we move out into a wider social world on our own initiative. Whether we leave this stage with a sense of initiative that outweighs our sense of guilt depends in large part on how parents respond to our self-initiated activities. Erikson emphasizes that this is the stage in which we begin to develop self-understanding, which is the representation of our emerging self.

Middle Childhood

In middle childhood, the latency period develops so that either a strong sense of industry and competence or a sense of inferiority sets in. As we move on to this stage of development, our attention focuses on being accepted by our peers and mastering tasks of a social nature: how well we fit into our social groups, the degree of comfort we feel, our degree of self-confidence, and the success we experience in school. If we fail to develop this important task we may develop social anxiety, social fears, and social isolation.

Puberty

Puberty marks the beginning of our transition into adulthood. We make this shift physically much more quickly. All of the tasks mastered up to this point in our development paved the way for this transition. The bonding and trust we learned in infancy provide the security we need as we risk relating to the opposite sex. This is the time when our emotions and our bodies are at odds. It is the time when we are most self-conscious physically and yet the most compelled to take emotional risks. The tension between our emotional and physical developments is what makes us feel so hopelessly awkward at this stage. No matter how old we are, there is no way through these feelings but to realize and deal with them, since they are directly connected to our self-esteem and our fears of not being accepted.

Adolescence

Adolescence marks the beginning of our transition into adulthood. Defining a self is the primary task in this developmental stage, which could be characterized by confusion, rebellion, and stress. For example, our adolescent self may rebel if we feel judged or intruded upon. We might rebel against authority figures, against the norm, or against social restrictions. Remember, rebelling is essential here in order to move successfully into adulthood. Adolescence is a time for the identity that becomes the foundation of our adult personality to form.

Ego identity and a sense of belonging regarding our careers, social roles, and sex roles develop or a crisis and role confusion sets in.

7

Ego identity, or identity confusion, sets in motion the directions in which our lives will proceed. Possessing a strong sense of identity, knowing who we are, having inner direction, developing inner strength, and having a strong sense of awareness, independence and compassion are all basic personality traits needed for achieving our fullest potential in adulthood.

Both Abraham Maslow (1962) and Carl Jung (1968) intensely studied this period of development. Maslow describes this process of self-awareness as "self-actualization," becoming everything we are capable of becoming. Jung describes this process as a journey to our unique self. He called it "individuation," becoming what we were destined to become. But for this process to fully succeed, we need to let go of many beliefs that might have served us well in the past but hinder our development today. Both Maslow's and Jung's belief that our purpose in life is to uncover our unique individual inner self which is an active process of becoming familiar with it by looking deeply inside and making that which is unconscious conscious.

Early Adulthood

As we proceed into adulthood we need to make clear distinctions between different sub-stages within this long lifecycle. The first stage of development in adulthood is early adulthood. It begins in our twenties and extends into our late thirties. Young adulthood is when we start being treated as adults. Learning how to be responsible, self-directed, motivated, focused, committed, and able to manage our time effectively are important issues to master at this stage of development.

Our goals become more concrete as we begin to discover what we want from life and make plans to achieve these goals. But for some of us it's not that simple, and we might regress to an earlier stage of development (i.e., adolescence) by acting out, procrastinating, remaining financially dependent, having difficulty keeping a job, and mismanaging money or time.

The messages that society conveys to us at this point in our lives are generally positive. Society encourages us to view this period as an opportunity for self-discovery, exploration, learning, and growth. The messages are "Challenge yourself to grow, to learn new things and to determine what fulfillment and authenticity mean to you. Experience different relationships, jobs, lifestyles and explore all available possibilities."

At this stage of life our intimate relationships are cemented, families are formed, careers are developed, interests are pursued, and new ventures are discovered. By twenty, we are confronted with questions, such as "How do we establish ourselves in the adult world?" "How do we put our aspirations into effect?" "How do we shape our dreams, which will generate energy, aliveness and hope?" Doing what we think we "should" or "what we are supposed to be doing" is the most pervasive theme of our twenties and thirties.

By our thirties, we have an idea of how our life is shaping up. Important new choices must be made in order to move on with our inner push for development. Life becomes more rational and orderly in our thirties, whether we decide to put down roots by getting married, having children, buying a home, climbing career ladders, or putting everything on hold to pursue a dream or hobby.

By our late thirties and early forties we are passing through a new crisis that gives us the window of opportunity to rework our identity. Many times this could cause us a full blown authenticity crisis. In order to come through this crisis, we must reexamine our purpose: Why are we doing the things that we are doing? What do we really believe in? Regardless of what we are doing today, these questions need to be addressed and dealt with.

Early-Middle Adulthood

The second stage of adulthood is early-middle adulthood, extending from our forties into our late fifties. This stage of development is a new space that has opened up since our life spans have been extended. It is a new pathway through the life course, a second and different kind of adulthood that precedes old age. This stage is a transitional period between young adulthood and middle adulthood, similar to our adolescent years, which served us as a transitional age between our childhood and young adulthood.

The physiological changes of adolescence that seem to trigger an intensified search for a sense of identity are mirrored by the physiological changes of aging. Just as in adolescence we grapple with the question of who we are, in early-middle adulthood we are faced with the same question: Who am I and what's happening to my body and mind? In adolescence we struggle to shape our personality. In early-middle adulthood we are trying to discard some of our assigned roles. We are confused in adolescence by the flood of hormones and confused again as they dwindle; confused in adolescence to discover acne on our faces and confused again to deal with wrinkles; confused to have been an object of sexual desire and confused again to become invisible.

These physiological changes are accompanied by social changes as we suddenly encounter a new set of attitudes and expectations and must grow into new roles. There may have been times when our parents said, "Act your age." Now, shockingly, our children may begin to say it. Our drive to combine our past and present, our inner life and public self, energizes the future with the promise of a growing sense of integrity and authenticity. As we begin to adjust to the notion that we are not who we were only older, we can imagine that what life is offering us is a chance to experience an entire transformation, i.e. anim-morphosis.

Early-middle adulthood could be called our second adolescence. For many women early- middle adulthood is a time of identity formation, of developing their sense of belonging regarding careers, new social roles, and sex roles. It's a time of exploration and commitment, as well as a time of great confusion. This age group women are not expected to be rebellious, but many times they are which is looked upon as childish and unbecoming. Nonetheless, rebellions are real and need to be dealt with at whatever age they resurface.

An "Aha!" moment may awaken us to a dormant self who was left unattended in the rush to make early choices. Too often the need for renewal is not acknowledged until we fall on our faces. Those who have taken risks through change and made one or more successful life passages are more likely to welcome the challenge to renovate their goals in early midlife or even beyond. Having reaped the benefits of purposeful change before, they will feel freer to shape a new self if they so choose to.

Although we all experience changes as we age—changes such as career development, marriage, or children—the visual image of ourselves remains relatively stable for much of adulthood until we enter into our early-mid adulthood and visible changes in our appearance occur. To be able to deal with these changes, we first need to mourn our youth and embrace the new stage of life that unfolds before our eyes.

In her book, *Motherless Daughters,* Hope Edelman (2004) describes the process of letting go and moving further toward the new. "No doubt, since our popular culture celebrates youth we are filled with fear and anxiety of our aging faces and bodies. The complex meaning behind exiting from our youthful self-image is a critical psychological experience that has to be embraced with courage. To leave the past behind and embrace the future takes courage and perseverance of the greatest kind. Most of us ascribe to the mantra: one day I will have a house, a partner, a different job, more money, or loose ten pounds. But at this point in our lives there is no later, only now – the present. Our time is running out and we need to do something about it" (129).

Early middle age is a time for an intense dialogue with ourselves: free of guilt, remorse and self-doubt. In this stage, life becomes more harmonious. We begin the search for our own authenticity. No one can dictate to us any more; we are in charge of our own lives. We can do what we want to do and enjoy our lives in the way we really desire. We are older, smarter, and more experienced so we are able to revisit all those roles that served us well in the past to see if they still work or if we need to make adjustments. This is our time. We might be facing new challenges, new possibilities, and new visions, but we are well prepared with an abundance of knowledge which we acquired through our fifty years of living.

For many women this milestone can be a time of self-reflection, which is a truly powerful experience. It may be a time to sit with the ever-nagging question—"Am I where I want to be?"—and come to peace with where we are. Or it might be a time to realize that there are many steps that haven't been taken, roads as yet unexplored, and there may be a need to make strong commitments to move forward in the coming years.

It takes courage to look within, but this is what we must do. By examining ourselves closely and coming to a deeper understanding of what matters most to us as unique individuals, we can separate social messages from our own hearts' calling and let go of ideas of "what should be" and instead embrace "what is."

Middle Adulthood

The third stage of development in adulthood is middle adulthood, which takes place from one's fifties to late sixties. Erikson called it "the age of generativity," and he saw this stage of development as a work in progress, a phase as momentous in character building as adolescence. With effort, self-determination, and self-awareness anyone could work toward a more meaningful life. Middle age encompasses productivity, creativity and further identity development.

This is the stage when we reflect on what we have done with our lives and all that we have accomplished so far. This is a good time for evaluating our lives and deciding if we need to change course. The doorway to this stage of life is filled with wisdom, opportunities, and a greater sense of freedom. For many of us this is a time to go back to school, change careers, develop new habits and relationships. It is not just that we are living longer, but our quality of life has improved because of better health care and more awareness about diet, exercise, nutrition, and mental wellness.

In our early-middle adulthood, we were defined by our relationship with others, whether it was our husbands, partners, or children. Most women identify themselves in terms of others; they think of themselves as daughters, mothers, wives. A major shift in women's development takes place in middle adulthood. Women move from dependence to greater independence. Women begin to see themselves as whole people with their own rights, separate from others. They tap into their originality of thought, sharpen their instrumental and critical skills, and master the complex environments where they now hope to operate.

Mastery is an accumulated inner strength, which is not dependent on immediate outer conditions or the approval of others. It's an inside job. What do we need to move toward mastery? First, we need to mourn our early-middle adulthood. We need to psychologically die before a new self can be born, before "anim-morphosis" can take place. We need to celebrate the dying of youth and stumble into the infancy of our mid-adulthood years. We need to break ourselves down before we can build ourselves up and reinvent ourselves.

The important attributes that we need to acquire on our road to mastery are resilience and self-mastery. Both of these attributes help us develop a deeper appreciation for the enormous complexity of human life. They will open doors to new learning, new discoveries, and new passions. Our intrinsic reward is a return to a sense of playfulness, curiosity, and a sharp edge of uncertainty. One simple rule is not to take ourselves too seriously. We must loosen up, or, as my grandchildren have repeatedly told me, "Chill out."

Late-Middle Adulthood

Openness and flexibility are important attributes during both our middle adulthood and our late-middle adulthood, which extends from our late sixties to our mid seventies. Not all of us are open to change. Some of us are stuck in the mode called "life prevention." This lack of openness to change restricts our actions and the possibility of new surprises that life has in store for us. Instead of trying to maximize control over our environment, which might have worked earlier in life, what works now is greater appreciation and acceptance for that which we cannot control.

We have reached a certain plateau in our family and career building. It's no longer necessary to invest all our energy in keeping up a "false self" to please and impress others. At this juncture in our lives, we can create a "new self" that beams with curiosity and adventurousness and is ready to embrace new discoveries, new learning, and roads not explored.

In his play *The Broken Glass*, Arthur Miller writes about a woman who gives up her career to accommodate her husband and family. In her fifties she develops a sudden hysterical paralysis in her legs. She returns to an infantile condition that puts her safely beyond any possibility of change. Unlike this woman's life circumstances, this stage is not a time to give up, but to actively find new values in life. The secret to finding meaning at later stages in our lives is to find our passions and pursue them with confidence in our abilities and strong convictions that we will succeed.

This book identifies what differentiates fulfilled, vital women from women paralyzed by fear at this juncture in their lives. Women with vitality have made the transitions in their thirties, forties, fifties, and sixties with a sense of freedom and optimism, a heartfelt openness to life's unpredictability, and a level of comfort with themselves and their bodies. They were able to create a bridge between the old ways that governed their lives and incorporate new visions, new possibilities, and new wants and needs. They were able with hard work to pursue their present dreams and not be swamped by inaction.

Late Adulthood

By late adulthood, in our late seventies and eighties, a sense of ego integrity develops. Here our wisdom rests in our capacity to see, look, remember, make decisions, and listen based on knowledge, experience, and insight accumulated over years. It seems logical that wisdom increases with age. The famous saying "becoming older and wiser by the day" is an appropriate phrase, but not always true.

Integrity demands tact, contact, and touch. It takes a lifetime to be tactful and demands both patience and skill or else we become weary and discouraged. It is a serious challenge in our mid eighties just to locate misplaced keys. Acceptance of one's life and the meaningful attributes accomplished throughout one's lifecycle is important. We must take responsibility for what our lives have been and become reconciled with our past as well as our future. We need to reward these years, or otherwise they get lost.

We can construct our own measure of life satisfaction. We can take pleasure in whatever round of activities constitutes our everyday lives, and we can hold a positive self-image regardless of what our present weakness may be. If this sense of integrity is lacking, a sense of despair will develop and a fear of death and hopelessness will set in.

Thinking that aging is unchangeable creates expectations of decline and then acceptance when the decline happens. This is caused by how our thought patterns and attitudes set the stage for how we act and what we accept as we get older. Our feelings, good or bad, are the products of our thought. We think first, then we feel. Our emotions have a powerful impact on our aging. Positive emotions produce high levels of serotonin, the feel-good chemical, while negativity depresses those hormones, causing us to age much faster.

The fear of moving through the golden years, as many of us call them, comes from the misguided societal message that "productivity is our lives' essence" and "retirement is unproductive and holds little value." In a society where the basic interest is in profit, old age cannot be honored because real honor would undermine the system of priorities that keep this society functioning and running.

So what becomes imminent is segregation between the old and the young. Old people feel isolated from the rest of the society, as well as invisible. No one wants to hear what old people have to say, which is a big liability for our society since their knowledge, wisdom, and life experiences are all invaluable information which is lost. Old people in general are irrelevant in our "youth obsessed" society, and all their experiences are unused and therefore wasted.

While there is no magical potion that can make the complex transitions through our lifecycles any easier, one thing is clear: having a positive attitude filled with curiosity rather than judgments about where we are and what we have is an important first step. Cultivating curiosity can enrich our lives to a point where it is not just bearable but exciting, joyous, and fulfilling. Without a doubt, the landmark fiftieth birthday casts a long shadow over women's lives, as it engages us in internal conversations about physical appearance, sexuality, relationships, career expectations, physical health, parenting, and care of our aging parents.

Reading this book will help the reader open up conversations on many of these different topics and guide them toward a better understanding about achieving their highest potential as they progress through their lifecycles. Understanding how we age will help us leave our confusions about aging behind and get on with discoveries about what we can do to stay healthy and youthful at any age.

The Foundation of Adult Personality

Exercise I

A safe, nurturing, and trusting environment that we experience during infancy sets the foundation for our adult personality; find out if you experienced a sense of safety, nurturance, and trust in your environment as you were growing up. Answer the questions below in your notebook. Try to remember as many details as you can going all the way back to infancy, or to the age that you can remember.

Safety

Are you capable of asking for help, or do you feel uncomfortable and refrain from asking?

Do you feel you have the right to ask others to meet your needs? Whom do you feel the most comfortable asking?

Do you feel safe around people that you don't know?

Do you have close, intimate relationships? How comfortable do you feel in these relationships?

Nurturance

How comfortable do you feel with closeness (being touched, kissed, hugged)?

Do you take care of yourself?

What are some things that you do for yourself?

Do you take care of others close to you?

Trust

Do you trust yourself to take care of yourself?

Do you trust people or are you suspicious of other people's motives?

Do you have a hard time opening up to friends?

Do you trust your abilities?

Review your answers and try to gain some understanding of what is going on in your life. For example, look at the group of statements under "Safety." Do you feel that you have issues with safety, like asking for help when you need, or do you have difficulty forming close relationships. What about nurturance and trust? If you don't perceive any big problems, then your caretakers probably met your basic needs and were physically affectionate. If you show signs that you have problems around nurturance, then your caretakers may not have been very affectionate. If your answers are extremes (always or never), that could indicate a lack of flexibility or a need to be in control. Use your own judgment to interpret the significance for you.

CHAPTER II

Enhancing Your Mind-Body Connection

"The body is an instrument, the mind its function, the witness and reward of its operation."

George Santayana

Our bodies will inevitably change, but our minds may not necessarily—at least to the degree which we expect. Our mind holds the most power over our body, and our body holds the most power over our mind. Our mind and body are one unit. When our body tells us that it is in need of something and our mind refuses to listen, imbalance begins, and the root of our mind-body connection is disrupted. For example, when we are tired and we need rest but our mind overrides this need in order to go out for dinner with friends, the disruption can throw us off. The same thing happens when our body needs to eat and our mind insists we work through lunch. Listening to the signals from our body and honoring them sets the stage for a healthy and well balanced body-mind interaction.

On the other hand, we can change our biology by what we think and feel. It would be impossible to isolate a single thought or feeling that does not have some effect on aging. Research has proven time and time again that stress, anxiety, despair, and depression all accelerate the aging process because those feelings raise our risks of heart attacks, high blood pressure, diabetes, obesity, or bulimia. On the other hand joy, fulfillment and stress reduction keep us healthy for longer. This means that the line between biology and psychology cannot really be drawn with any certainty. The mind and body are one unit that is indistinguishable.

Our beliefs, thoughts, and emotions fuel every cell in our body. They either energize our cells or deplete them of energy. Understanding how our thoughts and emotions effect every hormone and cell in our bodies and knowing how to change them in a way that is health enhancing gives us access to the most powerful health-creating secret. Natural foods, supplements, meditation, and exercise are all powerful tools for building and protecting our health. But even more important are our attitudes, beliefs, and daily thought patterns. How many times have we heard someone say, "I don't understand it. She always ate right and exercised. How come she got sick?" The answer lies at least in part in the individual's attitudes and emotions. Our attitudes, emotions, and beliefs can even influence how well our food is digested, how soundly we sleep, and how much benefit exercise brings.

We are capable of changing our world and body by simply changing our perceptions. How we perceive ourselves causes changes in our bodies. For example, the anthropologist Margaret Mead (1950) found in her research that in African societies where aging is accepted as part of the social fabric, elders remain vigorous. The decline of vigor as we age is largely the result of people expecting decline. To despair over growing old makes us grow old faster.

In order to stay alive, our bodies are in constant flux. For example, the skin replaces itself once a month, the stomach lining every five days, the liver every six weeks, and the skeleton every three months. To the naked eye, organisms look the same, but really they're constantly changing. By the end of each year, 98% of the atoms in our body will have been exchanged for new ones. Our bodies are not mindless machines; they are infused with a deep awareness of our needs.

Scientists have concluded that specific patterns of emotional vulnerability affect specific organs or systems of the body. There are dozens of medical studies on breast cancer showing that feeling powerless in important relationships and an inability to express emotions raise the risk of developing breast cancer. Similarly, studies have suggested that difficulties in handling negative emotions, especially hostility, are linked to heart attacks. Likewise feelings of hopelessness and helplessness can affect the immune system and increase susceptibility to infection and autoimmune diseases.

In the 1970s, the pioneering work of Hans Selye on stress and the mind-body connection was not accepted by mainstream society. He found that stress caused by frustration or prolonged emotional upset can cause physical harm. The physical results often take the form of psychosomatic illness, meaning bodily ailments.

Dr. Selye further emphasized that it's not stress that harms us but rather distress. Distress occurs when we prolong emotional distress and don't deal with it in a positive way. He referred to our bodies' response to stress as the "general adaptation syndrome" (G.A.S), which consists of three stages: the alarm stage, or the "fight or flight" response; the resistance stage, in which we adjust our bodies to counteract the physiological changes that occur in response to stress; and the exhausting stage in which the body actually creates the situation of distress.

These results were later substantiated by Joan Miller (1976) who found that people with high-stress jobs have a greater frequency of having ailments such as high blood pressure, stomach ulcers, and diabetes. In later years these researchers' compelling results were proven scientifically accurate, but at the time our culture simply was not ready for these ideas. We middle-aged women are ready, and we have the perfect opportunity right now to embrace this knowledge for ourselves while also sparking a fire of change in our culture at large.

A basic philosophy that I adopt in this chapter is that our physical and mental health depend more upon our perception of events surrounding us than upon the actual event, which means that our beliefs about our lives' events are more important than the events themselves. This is a truth that our culture does not teach. Instead, we are taught from an early age that our health is largely the result of our genetic heritage. We focus on whether or not we've been immunized, how many supplements we take, and how much we exercise. There is no doubt that all these factors are important contributors to our state of health, but their influence pales in comparison to the power of our beliefs and attitudes.

Letting go of the assumption that our bodies age because that is the way nature intended is an important first step. We need to relinquish the perceptions that have disabled us. If we accept that becoming old is inevitable, then we become victims. On the other hand, if we view getting old as something learned, we are in the position to unlearn these behaviors and adopt new beliefs that create new opportunities. If we are locked into the old paradigm that teaches us that old age is natural, painful, and inevitable, then our lives will be out of our control, and misguided, old assumptions will guide us. We need to challenge the way that we have been taught to understand the concept of aging and its causes.

Life in mid-middle adulthood, like in all other stages of development, could be measured by our chronological age (how old we are on the calendar), our biological age (how old our bodies are in terms of critical life signs), or by our psychological age (how old we feel). Our chronological age is the most unreliable, since a fifty-year-old may look like a thirty-year-old or a sixty-year-old. Our biological age is also a limited measurement of age. From a purely biological perspective, the aging process moves at such a slow rate that its fatal effects rarely match those of faster-moving diseases. Most critical organs can function well at thirty percent of peak capacity. Our biological age can be changed by such measures as regular exercise and good eating habits. We could lower our high blood pressure or excess body fat, and regulate sugar imbalances by treating our bodies well.

The greatest predictor of our aging process is our concept of our psychological age. Our calculation of our psychological or mental age is individualized. How old we feel has no boundaries. It's our personal choice. Research shows that biological age responds to psychological age. The saying, "You are as old as you think you are," certainly applies.

Changing our psychological age means adopting new ways of thinking, being, and believing. Additionally we need to incorporate into our lives regular daily work, job satisfaction, healthier relationships and friendships, control over our personal lives, enjoyable leisure time, hobbies, optimism about our futures, financial security, and living within our means. By nurturing our inner lives, we are using the power of awareness to defeat aging at its source. When we lean more towards negative emotions of apathy, hopelessness, and dissatisfaction, we push our bodies into rapid decline and accelerate the aging process.

Our body is the river of life, source of knowledge, and the fountain of information that sustains us. If we sit and listen to our bodies, we will find that a powerful intelligence dwells within them. We have to want to connect with our bodies before we can learn from them. We must be willing to open ourselves up to knowledge that we overlooked before.

Everything that has happened to us is recorded in our bodies and new possibilities await us as well. We often view aging as something that is happening to us when in fact it is something our bodies have learned to do. Our body carries out the programming that is fed into it by us, the programmers. Since so much of this programming is unconscious and dictated by our beliefs and assumptions, we do not always realize the effects of our input.

The first step towards experiencing our bodies in a different way is to change our perspective. Try letting go of the assumption that our bodies are aging because that is what nature intended. It's scary and difficult to erase imbedded thought patterns. However, we might need to replace them or modify them with new fresh ideas and challenges to accommodate our present needs.

The greatest enemy of renewal is habit. When old interpretations from the past are applied to the present, there will always be a mismatch between the needs of the moment and the solutions from the past. What we need is a willingness to allow ourselves to experience new visions and new perceptions which give rise to new solutions. But how do we accomplish this important task? First, we need to unfreeze the perceptions that have locked us into inaction by getting in touch with our body-mind connection. Awareness is the first step toward creating a healthy balance between our body and mind.

During early childhood, we are most impressionable. Our awareness is like fresh wax unhardened by experience. As we move through our life stages the same awareness becomes conditioned time and time again, and our minds become stiff. Aging bodies reflect this underlying rigidity which is felt in every cell of the body. The effect of conditioning is powerful, and choices become restricted.

For each of us, the learning process that teaches us to age is complex and never ending. It involves attitudes passed along from family, friends, and society since infancy. For example, what did your mother say when she saw her first wrinkles? Did she see them as dreaded symbols of lost youth? Or did she pay little attention? If we believe that we must age, then our bodies will conform to this conviction. If we inherit the expectation that our body must wear out over time, it brings about the biological phenomenon we call "aging," which in turn causes a great deal of physical and psychological distress.

All distress is simultaneously physical, psychological, emotional, and spiritual. What this means is that our entire body feels and thinks. Thoughts create feelings, and feelings create physical reactions. Our thoughts become words, then actions, and then habits. Our habits become who we are. A thought held too long will become a belief. The belief then becomes our biology. Beliefs are vibrational forces that create the physical basis for our individual lives and health.

If we don't work through self-destructive thoughts and subsequent feelings, our destructive thoughts set us up for physical distress because of the biochemical effects that emotions have on our immune system. For example, diseases such as rheumatoid arthritis or certain thyroid diseases are called autoimmune diseases because the immune system attacks the body. But it's not stress itself that creates immune system problems; rather, it's the thought that nothing can be done to prevent or change it. These negative thoughts are associated with immune system suppression. The good news is that our perceptions can always be changed, and that is the key to getting and staying well.

If we accept that our bodies are influenced by our thoughts and beliefs, that every thought is accompanied by an emotion or feeling, that every emotion creates a specific biochemical reality in our bodies, then it becomes clear that thoughts that are reinforced over and over become beliefs. Beliefs drive our behavior.

We inherit many of our beliefs from our parents and the circumstances of our upbringing. It is also important for us to understand that our beliefs go much deeper than our thoughts. Many beliefs are unconscious and are not readily available to the intellect. Sigmund Freud, the greatest psychologist of our time, stated in 1913 that both conscious and unconscious, negative and positive beliefs have equal influence on our bodies. Even things that we aren't aware of influence our physical and mental well-being.

In his book *Emotionally Free*, David Viscott (1993) makes the argument that through the years we store feelings as emotional debt, an action which is directly connected to aging. When we have emotional debt, we are pessimistic about our future. He identified a cycle of emotions that begins in the present, when only pain and pleasure are felt, and ends with complex feelings centered in the past, such as guilt and doubt. Pain in the present is experienced as hurt, pain in the past is remembered as anger, pain in the future is perceived as anxiety. This cycle of emotions operates continuously, generating both physical and psychological symptoms. Stored hurt is responsible for a wide range of psychological symptoms such as stress, anxiety, eating disorders, and insomnia.

Our bodies are designed to act as a receiving and transmitting station for energy and information. This simply means that we need to listen to our bodies and use our inner guidance that directs our thoughts and feelings to help us make conscious changes in our lives. Some of the messages that our inner guidance provides us with are positive messages.

There are many positive messages that we tell ourselves: "Our behaviors are based on our respect for ourselves and others." "There are many paths to joy." No one being is more superior to others." "Live in the moment." "Accept yourself and accept others." "Love yourself and take care of yourself." But there are plenty of negative messages as well: "Be selfish." "Be perfect." "Be better than everyone else." "Rehash the past with no future plans."

Frequently with these types of negative messages, we lose our creativity, our humor, and our laughter in pursuit of adult-like behaviors. Without humor one's thought processes are likely to become stuck, leading to distress and the harmful effects that distress has on our bodies and minds. We need to be aware, acknowledge, and accept our thoughts, feelings, and emotions without making judgments about them. We need to stop and stay with our thoughts—even those that might be painful or uncomfortable.

Accepting ourselves with all our feelings, positive and negative, is the first step on our road to mind-body anim-morphosis, or self-change. Often our healthy thoughts are trapped under irrational beliefs. As a result, we perceive things inaccurately by assuming, guessing, interpreting, or reading between the lines. Most of our fears and panic stem from our irrational thinking: thoughts that have no foundation, thoughts that aren't evaluated, thoughts that are mostly emotional in nature, or thoughts that are not well thought out.

The problem with this type of distorted thinking is that it has a negative impact on our bodies as well as on our psyches. Anxious thoughts create anxious feelings which create physical symptoms such as heart problems, ulcers, high blood pressure, hypertension, insomnia, and a general sense of restlessness.

All distortions or irrational thinking are actually bad habits. They are habits of thought that we constantly use to interpret reality in an unreal way. They are based on deeply held unrealistic beliefs and can cut us off from reality. Distortions are judgmental. They automatically apply labels to people and events before we get a chance to evaluate them. Therefore, distortions tend to be inaccurate. They allow us to see only one side of an experience, which gives us an unbalanced view of the world.

Finally, distortions are based on emotions rather than on rational thinking. Whenever an upsetting event occurs, automatic thoughts run through our minds. Although we are each capable of thinking reasonably about upsetting events, sometimes our automatic thoughts take over. These thoughts appear so fast that we hardly notice them or stop to question them. Yet these thoughts profoundly affect our moods and our sense of worth. That's why it's essential for us to examine some of our most frequently held irrational beliefs.

Challenge Your Irrational Thinking

The most frequently held irrational thoughts are black or white thinking, emotional reasoning, generalization, controlling, self-blaming or other-blaming, and minimizing the good while maximizing the bad.

Black or White Thinking: It's either bad or good, with nothing in between. For example, you are on a diet, and you eat a spoonful of ice cream. Then you tell yourself, "I've blown my diet completely." This thought might be so upsetting that you decide to gobble down an entire quart of ice-cream. This type of thinking does not allow for shades of gray. You judge yourself as either good or bad, a success or a failure. Reinterpret the same event with rational thinking: "I ate a spoonful of ice cream. It's ok. I needed it to calm my nerves after a long day. Tomorrow I will go back to watching what I eat. I can give myself permission to indulge when I feel the need to do so."

Global Thinking or Generalization: A small thing becomes a universal event. You see a single negative event, such as a friend's rejection, as a never ending pattern of defeat. For example, you might say, "I always get rejected by my friends. No one likes me. everybody hates me." To fight this type of irrational thinking, you need to get rid of absolute terms such as "all," "every," "none," "everybody," "never," "always" and so on. You need to accept that some people will approve of you and some won't. You need to be a healthy optimist. Expect to find small ways to improve situations and notice what is going well.

Minimizing the Positive: Rejecting positive experiences and insisting they don't count. You selectively extract certain facts from reality and pay attention to them, ignoring all the rest. For example, someone compliments your dress. You reply, "Oh it's nothing. It's just an old dress." You could have just as easily replied, "Thank you." You have blind spots that obscure evidence of your own worth and dismiss the good as not important.

Emotional Reasoning: Assuming negative emotions reflect the way things really are. Here you believe your negative feelings without questioning them. For example, a friend may not call you, and you think, "My friend didn't call me. She must be angry with me, or she found other friends and dropped me." This type of emotional reasoning is based on feelings instead of rational laws. You rely on emotions to interpret reality. To fight this you need to create self-rebuttals that omit emotionally charged words like "love," "hate," "furious," depressed, and so on.

Self Blame and Other Blame: Your hold yourself personally responsible for an event that is not entirely under your control. For example, you might think, "My child misbehaved in school. This shows that I'm a bad mother." Your child's behavior is partly under your control, but not completely. You can't take full blame. Other blaming is the opposite: you blame others for your problems and put all responsibility on someone or something outside of yourself. For example, you might think of someone, "He makes me so mad," or "I'm a loser because of my crummy upbringing." The problem with blaming others is that it tends to make you think of yourself as a helpless victim. The world is not totally under your control, but it's not out of your control either.

Controlling: Giving a false feeling of omnipotence. You struggle to control every aspect of every situation. You hold yourself responsible for your behavior and those of others. For example, you may think to yourself, "I've got to make them listen" in a situation where you're not really in control. Your rebuttal must emphasize your actual and real control over your life and nothing more.

Shoulds, Musts, Oughts: These are all demands you make of yourself. Here are some common ones: "I should be a perfect lover." "I must not make mistakes." "I should know better." You think that you motivate yourself with such statements. Usually, though, you just feel worse, frustrated, ashamed, and hopeless. One solution is to replace "should" with "would," "could" or "want." For example, "It would be nice if I did that," "I wonder how I could do that," or "I want to do that because it's to my advantage—not because someone is telling me I should."

Catastrophizing: Blowing things out of proportion. Catastrophizing imagines that the worst is going to happen or makes negative predictions in your mind. Try to ask yourself what evidence you have to support negative views that the worst will happen, what you can do to decrease the prospect of it happening, and, in case it happens, what you can say to yourself to cope.

Self-Downing: Being extremely critical of yourself is one of the most frequently used types of irrational thinking. Here you continually put yourself down. For example, you think, "I'm not good at any sports," "I'm such a failure," or "I'm stupid for saying those things to my friend." Now ask yourself what would a good friend say to you at this moment? Try to reframe the negative thoughts to reflect the positive in the situation.

Consider two scenarios. Imagine for a moment you overhear a conversation between a teacher and a student. A student is struggling with a math problem, and you hear the teacher say to the student: "You are so lazy, you didn't even try to figure out the problem yourself." Or you're at a playground, and a child falls off the slide and the mother comes running over to the child and says. "You're so clumsy. I can't believe you fell." How would you respond to hearing these types of critical, judgmental, and blaming statements directed at a young child in despair?

Answer these two questions in your notebook and examine the feelings that the statements evoked in you. Do you find it easier to be compassionate to strangers? If the answer is yes, then examine why. And if the answer is no, it means that you treat yourself as you treat others, meaning if you're critical of yourself you will be critical of other as well. If you're compassionate with yourself, you will be compassionate to others as well.

To combat distorted thinking you must master the most important skill: honest self-awareness. You must constantly listen to what you tell yourself. Take any of your major and frequently reoccurring irrational beliefs, and spend a few minutes every day disputing them. Write them down in your notebook. Here are some samples.

Negative thought: Why am I always late for work? I'm so disorganized. I have a problem with time management. My boss must think that I'm a failure.

Positive thought: It's true that time keeping is not my strongest attribute, but I can start managing my time more effectively. Just because I'm late sometimes does not mean that I'm useless. The feedback I get from my job and friends shows that I am highly regarded.

You might also use a reward system after you spend time disputing your irrational thoughts. Select an activity which you enjoy, and use it as a token or treat. For example, give yourself permission to do something that you enjoy like go to the movies or go shopping.

Challenge Exercise I
Replacing Your Irrational Thoughts with Rational Ones

Step 1: Identify your activating event. Lauren needs to give an oral presentation for her English class. She forgets to make some points she had intended to. However, no one in her class, including the teacher, noticed. At the end of her presentation students were asking her interesting questions which she answered well.

Step 2: Irrational thought: "My presentation was useless. The teacher did not make enough positive commends." Feeling: Lauren is frustrated at herself.

Step 3: Replace it with a rational thought: "Some students looked interested and ask good questions. The teacher made some good observations. I might not have included everything I wanted in my presentation, but there is no real evidence to suggest that anyone thought I didn't do a good job." Give yourself permission to make mistakes. No one is perfect all the time. Allow yourself to learn from your mistakes as much as you learn from your successes.

Step 4: Record your rational thought: "I give myself permission to make mistakes. No one is perfect all the time."

Summary

Be aware of the fact that all negative feelings are a result of your negative thinking. When you're unhappy or anxious, you probably think about something bad that happened to you. This phenomena is natural when bad things happen. But many times your thoughts go toward irrational thinking without anything bad happening to you. These are the type of thoughts that you have to be aware of and create an arsenal of rebuttals to combat. As the Greek philosopher Epictetus said, "Men are not disturbed by things, but the view they take of them."

Learn how to replace your negative thoughts with reality-based thinking. Set yourself free from irrational thoughts that run your life and make you miserable. Recognize which are your most frequent distortions. Familiarize yourself with the way you are using them. Catch them as they occur and put a stop to them by developing strong rebuttals. With knowledge, self-awareness, and motivation you can change your life's destiny. It's that easy.

By replacing negative thoughts with more objective reality-based thinking, you separate facts from fiction. You need to retrain your thinking. Like many other training programs, it takes time, repetition, and patience.

Obstacles

Some common obstacles which might prevent you from acknowledging your negative thinking are denial, overcompensation, and resignation.

Denial means simply denying that you have a problem. The best way to face up to denial is reflecting without shame on the situation. If you are ashamed of something, then one way of dealing with it is to deny that you have a problem. Addressing your shame-filled self-deprecation can help you admit to yourself that you have a problem. For example, "I know that I am very aggressive with my friends, and that's why most of them break up with me. This has been my problem for many years. Now I need to do something about it. I need to change my behavior and gain back my friends' trust."

Overcompensation is when you adopt a stance that is the very opposite of how you truly feel. The only problem is that this strategy only serves to reinforce the irrational belief that you are trying to overcompensate for. For example, "I'm going to do a good job even though I know that they don't deserve it."

Resignation is accepting the status-quo. You see yourself as lacking the possibility for change, or you say to yourself, "I'm okay the way I am." As a result, you resist the idea of self-acceptance, and you stay with your irrational beliefs without any possibility for relieving the stress that they may cause.

Remember, you need to hold constant vigilance over your thoughts so that you're able to stop your distortions when they occur. This simple awareness sets in motion the foundation for your body-mind connection. Being aware of your thoughts and being able to stop your distorted thinking and replace it with more realistic thinking are the keys that unlock the door to your mental and physical health. You now know that every thought and emotion you have fuels every cell in your body. Understanding how your thoughts effect every hormone and cell in your body and knowing how to challenge them by promoting both physical and mental health gives you important access to your mind-body interconnection. Understanding and acknowledging this connection promotes and protects your health and wellbeing throughout your life.

A healthy mind creates a healthy body, and a healthy body creates a healthy mind. Challenging your body-mind interconnection is central to your quest toward a better and healthier middle age. With your body strong and your brain sharper, you are ready to create for yourself the best life possible.

CHAPTER III

Psychological Anim-Morphosis
Reclaiming Your Authentic Self

"A person cannot be comfortable without their own approval."

Mark Twain

"Grant me the serenity to accept what I cannot change, the courage to change what I can, and the wisdom to know the difference."

Reinhold Niebuhr

While the previous chapter dealt with our body-mind inter-connection, the present chapter's main focus is on our self: our self-esteem, self-awareness, self-acceptance, self-understanding, self-appreciation, and self-love.

Since you make up your entire life's script, you are its author and editor. The type of life you are creating for yourself is all in your hands. Either you work for yourself, or you work against yourself. Either you are a true friend to yourself, or you are just going through life mindlessly letting things happen to you. You feel out of control, hopeless, helpless, and blame the world for all your misfortunes. This chapter's main purpose is to shed some light on this simple reality and the importance of living an authentic life, which can only be done with an authentic self, i.e. a real self. A false, pretend, fake, or idealized self will not do. But how do you know that you operate with a real self and not a false self?

First, you need to re-examine your old definitions, roles, and personality characteristics that defined you for the first fifty or sixty years of your life to see if those roles work for you today. If they don't, then learn new ways of being and living to achieve a healthier and more fulfilling life at middle age. You need to ask yourself: "How comfortable am I with my life today?" It would be sad to waste your energy on something that doesn't work well today and hinders your quality of health and wellness.

Now stop for a moment and imagine your life one year from now. If it's the same as it is right now, are you okay with that? If the answer is "yes," then congratulations. Whatever you're doing, keep doing it. But if the answer is "no," then my next question would be: "What would you want to be different and what are you doing to bring about these changes?"

Most of us want a change in at least one area of our lives, but we feel stuck. We don't know how to begin, or something keeps stopping us. That something could be fear, confusion, lack of awareness, low self-esteem, lack of guidance, or hopelessness. These obstacles make us think that our dreams are out of our reach. But as this chapter points out, we all have within us the power to change those things that don't work for us. All we need is self-awareness and guidance on how to achieve this important task.

Your Self Today

Before you continue reading further, here are two simple exercises that will serve as a starting point for how you feel about yourself at this time. These exercises will help you process the information in this chapter more easily and help you realize that you already have a self-esteem to build on.

Exercise I

Answer the following statements as honestly as you can. Rate yourself from 1 to 10 on how much you believe each of the following statements. One means you totally disbelieve it, and ten means you think the statement is totally true.

I respect myself.

I accept myself with both my negative and positive attributes.

I am good to myself.

I take care of myself, and I don't expect others to take care of my needs.

I can laugh at myself and make light of myself when needed.

I don't take myself too seriously.

I am happy to be me.

The lower your numbers are, the more work you need to do on your overall self. The higher the numbers are, the closer you are to having a good sense of self and of well-being.

Exercise II

Now examine the following questions to determine in which area you would like some guidance. When you finish reading this chapter, come back to these questions, re-examine them, and answer them again to see if the way you perceive and think of yourself has changed. And if so, pay attention to how those perceptions of yourself have changed.

How can I develop a healthy sense of self?

How can I learn to feel good about myself?

When I hear the world "high self-esteem" or "low self-esteem," what does it mean?

Can a person have too high of a self-esteem in one area of their lives and low self-esteem in other areas?

Is self-esteem based on looks or personality or both?

What are the consequences of having low self-esteem?

Can you recover from low self-esteem in middle age?

How can you develop unconditional self-acceptance?

Is unconditional self-acceptance being selfish?

Your Journey Toward Self-Discovery

The journey toward our self-discovery is both exciting and necessary in middle age. The more open and honest we become with ourselves, the more accepting and forgiving we will be—becoming a true partner to ourselves on this road toward self-rediscovery and change. We all make judgments about ourselves and others around us. Our judgments could come either from a positive place or from a negative one. Examples of negative judgment would be "I'm not smart enough," "I'm not pretty enough," or "I'm not good enough." This means that our self-esteem is very much connected with our self-perception and goes to the core of our identity. As a result, our core identity determines to what degree we see ourselves as worthy, smart, or loved.

Both positive and negative core beliefs formulate the rules we use in our daily lives. For example, when we tell ourselves that we cannot lose weight, we convince ourselves that's the truth, and we sabotage ourselves by overeating or by not paying attention to what or how much we eat, which results in weight gain. In this case, our prediction about ourselves has become a reality.

Our core beliefs are the foundation of our self-esteem. Expressed as our rules, they dictate what we can and cannot do. Expressed by our inner dialogue, they determine how we interpret events in our world. A negative core belief might be something like "I'm incapable of making good decisions" or "Every time I have to make a decision, I mess up." A positive core belief would be "I have good judgment when it comes to making decisions and even though sometimes it's not the best choice, it's okay. I can learn from all my decisions."

We all need to re-examine the old rules that governed our lives to see if they work as well today as they worked in the past. This can be done by getting in touch with our authentic self, the real self, and closely examining what our self needs today and what we are telling ourselves. Our authentic self represents our honest assessments of ourself—without lies, excuses, denials, or false pretense. When we eliminate all that is false, we are left with everything that is real. But the big question remains, do you want to know yourself? If your answer is "yes," keep reading.

I remember throughout graduate school and my career as a psychologist and professor, every time the concept of the development of self would arise, I would ask my students a simple question: "Who are you?" Most of their answers would pertain to their work, career, family, relationships, or even history, but very few were able to define themselves in terms of their individual personality traits. I realized that most of them did not understand my question. Yes, what you do is important, but there are many facets to a person in order to arrive at "you," or your authentic self.

So let's start this discovery of your authentic self by exploring a few important questions: Who are you? Do you ever stop and think of yourself? Do you know yourself? Why are you doing what it is you're doing? Does what you do reflect who you really are? Given a choice would you choose differently? Do you even know what you would choose? Wouldn't it be sad if a different, vibrant you was buried under the pile of worldly to-do list obligations and you were mindlessly accepting these expectations?

Your self is the you that can be found at your absolute core. It is all your unique strengths, values, gifts, skills, and wisdom that need expression, as opposed to what you have been programmed to believe about who you are "supposed" to be and what you are supposed to be doing. Living in a world with assigned roles rather than an authentic self drains you of the critical life energy you need to live well. In contrast, if you gain awareness and get in touch with your true, authentic self, then all that wasted life energy could be redirected toward a more fulfilling life.

This chapter is about letting go of mindless living and embracing mindfulness. It's about stopping the mindless performance of all the roles you would never choose but have been assigned. It's about getting in touch with your real self. It's about taking care of yourself. Most importantly, it's about accepting yourself. To do any less would be to cheat yourself physically, mentally, and emotionally. It takes a lot of energy to be what you are not, and it takes so little to be what you truly are.

If we begin to question who we are, then we don't have a solid foundation upon which to build our lives. If we don't know who we are, then how can we decide what's good for us or what to do? Having a strong sense of identity sets the foundation upon which we can build our lives. Without that foundation, our lives will disintegrate, haunted by fear, inaction, stress, anxiety, uncertainty, doubts and confusion.

In the previous chapter, I described in detail the development of our lifecycle. By the time we hit the early adolescent years (twelve to fifteen years of age), we start having a sense of identity. Adolescents wonder, "Who am I as an individual?" Erikson called the quest during this time "the search for identity." This quest for identity resurfaces all throughout our life. For the purposes of this book, I will concentrate on our quest for our identity through the three sub-phases of middle adulthood: early-mid adulthood, middle adulthood and late-middle adulthood.

Self-Esteem

Our behaviors, attitudes, values, and beliefs reflect the view we have of ourselves and the way we value the various parts of our personality. This is at the core of our self-esteem. Self-esteem is the component of personality that encompasses our positive and negative self-evaluations. Although we all have a general level of self-esteem, it's not one-dimensional. We may see ourselves positively in one area but negatively in other areas. For example, a woman may have high self-esteem in her career, but a lower self-esteem in her self-image.

In *The Principles of Psychology* (1890), the great psychologist William James defined self-esteem by a formula of success over pretensions. By pretensions he meant our aspirations or goals. In his view, self-esteem will increase if we are successful in achieving our goals, and it will increase even more if we achieve higher than we aspire to. His position was that if we don't succeed in reaching our goals, our self-esteem will suffer.

Following the same line of thought, I argue that in order to increase one's self-esteem, it's sensible to set realistic goals rather than overly optimistic ones. However, I would also suggest that we don't want to set our goals too low, or we may lose all motivation. It's about achieving a sensible balance. This kind of balanced approach to ourselves and our lives in general can be a more secure route to a reasonable level of self-esteem than focusing our attention exclusively on achieving success.

Self-esteem is a realistic and appreciative opinion of ourselves. "Realistic" in this case means honest, accurate, and open, while "appreciative" means accepting, positive, and loving. People whom we refer to as having an excess of self-esteem could be sometimes confused with those that have a self-defeating pride, meaning they try to be better than others. Usually they're arrogant, narcissistic, and think that they are better than anyone else around them. On the other end of the spectrum are people we refer to as having low self-esteem, or a self-defeating sense of self. These people hold an unrealistic and unappreciative opinion of themselves. Those are the ones that are critical, judgmental, and hold a very negative view of themselves and others.

Many of our problems are the direct or indirect result of how we feel about ourselves. It is a fact of life that we can never be any better than our own self-esteem. Thus, we can't exceed how we feel about ourselves in relation to others because that relation is based on our sense of self-acceptance. These feelings are basically unconscious and have been programmed into our subconscious since early childhood.

Positive self-esteem is not the intellectual acceptance of one's talents and accomplishments. It is personal self-acceptance. Developing positive self-esteem is not an ego trip. We simply realize that we are a truly unique and worthy individual, one who does not need to impress others with achievements, material possessions, or beauty. Developing positive self-esteem is not just a matter of making ourselves happy; it's the foundation on which we must build our whole lives.

Genuine self-esteem is not competitive or comparative. Neither is genuine self-esteem expressed by self-glorification at the expense of others. Arrogance, boastfulness, and the overestimation of our abilities reflect inadequate self-esteem rather than too high a level of self-esteem.

A person with high self-esteem possesses the ability to speak of accomplishments and shortcomings with honesty, to take criticism and be comfortable talking about mistakes, to express curiosity about new ideas and the possibilities in life. This person is also flexible and possesses the ability to see and enjoy the funny aspects of life in one's self and others. He or she is able to take compliments well, to be assertive when needed, to listen and cooperate well, and to give credit to others and to take constructive criticism. These are just a few of the attributes people with high self-esteem possess.

Although almost everyone goes through periods of low self-esteem, some of us are chronically low in self-esteem. For these people, failure seems to be an inevitable part of life. In fact, low self-esteem may led to a cycle of failure in which past failure breeds future failure. And eventually the failure reinforces low self-esteem. It becomes a vicious cycle that can hinder quality of life.

There are many reasons for someone to develop a low self-esteem, but the most important causes are developed in our early childhood years. They stem from a series of self-defeating concepts, beliefs, and values that we have accepted from our parents. By far the strongest single contributing factor to our faulty self-esteem is the low self-esteem imparted by our parents at a very young age.

Freud (1933) described the first six years of our lives as setting the foundation of our adult personality. If parents feel inadequate and inferior, we as children feel unworthy, and as a result we are unable to cope with even the simplest problems in home or school life. In essence, our parents' misguided concepts of self are the catalyst through which we develop a misguided concept of self. For example, when our parents told us that we were "bad," we misinterpreted this and felt that we were bad, when, in reality, only our actions were bad. The truth of the matter is that there is no such thing as a "bad child." The only thing "bad" about any child is the lack of awareness about what produces the best results.

Low self-esteem is further developed through the common habit of belittling by comparison. When parents compare a child with a sibling or someone outside the family, our own budding sense of inferiority is compounded. In the light of the flaws we have come to accept as part of our own make-up, we compare ourselves to children of the same age whom we admire. Believing that they are endowed with more ability, popularity, and self-confidence than we are, a devastating sense of inferiority sets in.

Lack of recognition and appreciation of individual uniqueness is another parental failing. Some parents pay little regard to their children's feelings, desires, and opinions, rebuffing them, often with the claim that mother or father knows best. These parents believe that their child alone has a problem when actually the problem is a mutual one involving both the parents and their offspring.

Many people with low self-esteem will fall prey to unhealthy addictions like overeating or alcohol consumption to numb their sense of inadequacy. The severity of addictions are a direct reflection of a person's sense of inadequacy and fear at having to justify who and what she is. The addicted person uses her alibi to cover up the low self-esteem she doesn't want others to see.

People with low self-esteem suffer a personal blow to their entire existence. They cannot cooperate or listen well. They are critical, judgmental, and they always see the bad in themselves as well as others. They can only talk of their accomplishments. They cannot take criticism. They're sensitive, and they have a weak ego. They're usually depressed, sad and unmotivated.

It is important for us to recognize that we will only be as happy and at peace with ourselves to the degree to which we accept the reality of the present frame of reference from which we are operating. Once we accept reality, we will no longer be vulnerable to the adverse opinions of others. Our refusal or inability to accept things as they are is at the root of our problem. Only when we can recognize a particular phase of reality for what it is at the present moment is our resistance to it lifted. If we are not conscious that we are resisting reality, there is no way for us to break this destructive habit.

Self-Awareness

Our first step in honoring ourselves and developing a healthy self-esteem is to choose to be conscious and self-aware. We must make the choice to think, to be aware of our outer world as much as our inner world. To honor the self is to be willing to think independently and to have the courage of our own perceptions. We also need to be willing to know not only what we think, but also what we feel, want, and need. The opposite of this attitude is denial, self-deprivation, self-stagnation, which means the general denial of "self."

To honor the self is to preserve an attitude of self-acceptance, which means accepting both our positive and our negative traits. Acceptance, without any pretense about the truth of our own being, is key. Pretense is aimed at deceiving either ourselves or others. To honor ourselves is to live authentically in the present, allowing us the possibility to grow and to discover our potential at any age during our lifecycle. Doing anything less would simply deny our own existence.

Our greatest barriers to growth and success are not lack of ability, but rather our inability to see what our abilities are. This is a lack of self-awareness. The great twentieth-century psychologist Carl Rogers (1961) pointed out that we only use a small amount of our potential and self-awareness throughout our life span. The rest goes to waste because we are not aware of its existence.

Our awareness can be defined as the clarity with which we consciously perceive and understand everything that affects our lives. It is the sum total of our life experiences, knowledge, intellect, intuition, instincts, and all that we perceive through our five senses. Our present level of awareness affects our moods, attitudes, emotional reactions, habits, desires, fears, aspirations, anxieties, and goals. Most importantly, it mirrors our sense of personal worth. In other words, it reflects how we feel about ourselves.

Awareness determines our concept of reality. Our mind is like a camera that is constantly taking pictures of the events in our lives. We are the ones who decide what kinds of scenes we wish to film or record, and these things make up our awareness. Let's remember: every decision we make and every action we take is based on our present level of awareness. The truth is that we can never be any better than we are at this moment because we are limited by our present level of awareness. And even if our best is faulty, to know better is not sufficient to do better. We will only do better when our "awareness" is closely examined, questioned, and expanded.

The first step that we need to take to expand our sense of awareness is to open a dialogue with our inner voice. What is our inner dialogue? This is the conservation that we have with ourselves about everything that's going on in our lives. Our inner dialogue is at the core of our being. It is the private dialogue that we have with ourselves that no one else is part of.

In time we become disconnected from our healthy inner voice because of abuse, criticism, or abandonment, and we conclude that were are flawed as individuals. We don't believe that we make mistakes but rather that we are all bad at our core. Thus, our inner voice becomes negative, and, as a result, we reject, judge, and criticize ourselves. This is at the root of self-hatred, dislike, shame, and rejection. The truth is that our inner voice can be healed. The cure is simply self-acceptance and self-love.

Here are some examples of unhealthy self-dialogue: "I must not make mistakes at my job because everyone will laugh at how stupid I am, including my boss." Or, "I can't lose weight, so I'm fat and ugly." Or "My friends treat me unfairly. They don't like me. I must be bad or just stupid for putting up with it." Replacing these types of self-defeating dialogues with healthy dialogues is our first step. But first, we need to become fully aware of what we are telling ourselves about ourselves. Specifically we need to pay attention to the words that we use to describe ourselves, such as stupid, bad, ugly, fat, and so on. A healthy self-dialogue would sound more like: "I wonder how I can do things differently next time." Or, "I wonder how I could change my eating habits to lose a few pounds. I need to came up with a better eating plan." Or, "It would be nice if my friends and I would develop a different type of relationship, but if we don't, it's okay; now, let me see what I can do to improve things with my friends."

The problem is that most of our internal dialogues are filtered. It is as if we have sunglasses over our internal dialogue. Some things we see; some we don't. Through these filters we process and assign a meaning to every event in our lives. Some things flow in while others are screened out. Whatever passes through the filter, accurate or not, is what we tend to believe and act on. As a result, if our filtered perceptions lie, we get stuck, and we believe in an upside-down world as being real. An example of a filtered inner dialogue would be "I always make mistakes. I'm so stupid." In contrast, an example of a healthy inner dialogue would be "I'm fine. I'm doing the best I can at this moment." As our healthy inner dialogue gains more power, it responds more quickly to the attacks of our filtered inner dialogue.

Now let's ask ourselves, why do we listen to a filtered inner dialogue that does not possess all the facts? First, we are familiar with our filtered inner dialogue because we have probably used it most of our adult lives. It keeps us secure by eliminating things that are frightening us. This voice helps us cope with feelings of anxiety, helplessness, and rejection. Paradoxically, while this filtered voice is beating us up, it also makes us feel better for the moment.

But we are paying a heavy price, and it undermines our self-worth. For example, a filtered inner voice might tell us "This relationship ruined my entire life," while an unfiltered voice might say, "Nobody, but me can ruin my life. I'm fully responsible for my own life." In this example it is clear that as long as we place the responsibility on the outside world without taking any blame for our actions or engage in irrational thought (in this case, other blaming), then we can't see any possibility of making changes within our lives, leaving us helpless and hopeless with the feeling that our life is out of our control.

This is where our internal dialogue can cause problems. For example, the internal dialogue for a person with low self-esteem can generate an excuse for playing it safe and not expecting too much from life. This kind of thinking can be seen in moments of self-dialogue such as "Everybody has doubts," "I'm not good with my hands, so I won't try playing any instrument, though I would like too," "I'm so disorganized with everything that I do in my life," or "I'm just plain stupid, that's why I have no friends."

We need to challenge our inner critic and not allow it to take over our lives. We need to become aware of what we are telling ourselves and replace our negative dialogue with a positive one. Positive internal dialogues are rational and optimistic and consist of thoughts, messages and facts that allow us to live in accordance with reality, not lies, assumptions, or excuses. A positive internal dialogue is a truthful engagement with the world and not smiley-faced denials. It is not about developing a litany of "feel good" mantras ("I'm good enough" or "I'm happy enough"), but having an honest conversation with ourselves about ourselves, which means talking about facts, not fiction or fantasy.

Nothing but candid truth will do. If our self-talk is filled with self-doubt, we will live that truth. But if our self-talk is confident and streetwise, we won't be fearful even in a high risk situation. Our reaction will be a result of what we perceive about ourselves. People with low self-esteem do not see themselves clearly. The image they see, like a reflection in a funhouse mirror, magnifies their weaknesses and minimizes their assets. To raise one's self-esteem it is absolutely necessary to throw away the old warped mirror and learn to accurately perceive one's particular balance of strengths and weaknesses.

Examine Your Self-Concept

Exercise III

This exercise will help you create a clear and accurate self-description. Instead of filtering out your strengths and magnifying your weaknesses, you can learn to recognize and value the person you really are. Let's start with an accurate self-assessment of yourself. Write down in as much detail as possible how you see yourself at the present time. Answer the following questions as accurately as you can. Start with a calming breathing exercise to get into a relaxed state of mind. Close your eyes, and breathe in and out. Breathe slowly and pay attention to the breathing rhythm. Notice and eliminate the tension that you might feel in different parts of your body. Notice where you feel tense in your body and focus on that place. Listen to the thoughts that go through your mind. Notice everything that you are saying to yourself and the feeling that it triggers. If your inner voice is saying something negative about what you're doing at the moment, recognize it, and try to see its function. It's trying to help you or hold you back. If it's trying to hold you back, then start talking back and make it useless. Tell it, "Stop it. Those were the things my teacher told me when I was six and they don't apply now. No more put downs. Stop this garbage." Once you're relaxed, answer the following questions.

How would you describe your physical appearance: your height, weight, facial appearance, skin, hair, style of dress, neck, chest, waist and legs?

How do you describe your mental ability: intelligence, creativity, learning, curiosity, interests and street smarts?

What are some of your personality traits (both positive and negative)?

How do you take care of yourself: hygiene, health, nutrition, physical activities, hobbies, vacations, fun time, food preparation, dressing, hair style and make-up?

How well do you reason and solve problems? What is your capacity for learning, creativity, special interests, wisdom, insights, and so on?

When you are finished answering these questions, go back and put a plus sign by items that represent strength and put a minus by items you consider weaknesses or would like to change. Don't mark items that are neutral or factual observations about yourself.

You just learned how you perceive yourself. You learned about your strengths and weaknesses and the areas in which these strengths and weaknesses are manifested. You may find that the vast majority of your minus items show up in just one or two areas of the inventory. If that's the case, your self-esteem is generally good, but you have a few specific weak spots. The more your minus items are spread throughout the inventory, and the larger the proportion of minus to plus items, the more effort it will take to achieve a realistically positive self-image.

There is nothing wrong in having faults. The problem is not having such a list but the ways in which you use your weaknesses for destructive self-attacks. Saying that you hide your anger with your friends is a reasonable assessment, but to condemn yourself as "phony with friends" undermines your self-esteem. There are four rules you need to follow when you begin revising the items on your list of weaknesses. First, use no pejorative language. Use accurate language. Use language that is specific rather them general. Finally, be kind to yourself.

A Conversation with Your Inner Voice

The next step on your road to self-discovery is opening up an honest dialogue with your internal voice. How does your internal voice operate? Your internal voice is affected by your core beliefs, and it helps to reinforce those beliefs. Your core belief and your inner dialogue are interconnected. If you tell yourself constantly that you are stupid, then you convince yourself that this is true. By the same token, if your self-statement reflects a basic faith in your intelligence, this core belief will be solidified. Remember, core beliefs are the foundation of your self-esteem, and they largely dictate what you can and cannot do and how you interpret events in your world.

It's hard to catch yourself in the act of thinking negative thoughts. Such thoughts can be so much a part of you that it becomes hard to sort them out from other background noise in your life. Get acquainted with your internal voice.

Describe Yourself

Exercise IV

What do you tell yourself about yourself?

1) Write down what you tell yourself about yourself: your body, your intelligence, your abilities and skills, your worth, your relationships, your values, your attitudes, and your moral standing.

2) Now imagine that you are going to your class reunion. All your friends will be there. It is the night before the reunion, and you are lying in bed in the dark. What are you saying to yourself? Write your thoughts down word by word.

Look through the answers to the questions above. Do you see common threads running through both sets of writing? If so, what are those common threads? Describe them in writing. What is the tone or mood of your internal dialogue? Is it positive, negative, or self-doubting? If it's positive, is it rational? Or is it a fantasy with no substance? Circle any writing that you think illustrates either positive or negative dialogues.

When mindless, unchallenging routines dominate there can be no authenticity and you are trapped in a descending circle of aimless existence. If you go through life as a robot you are not equipped to play the game of life well. The only reason you are holding on to your past habits is that you have not created new habits to replace them. You need to be in a place where you refuse to sell out your dreams and visions and start getting in touch with your authentic self of today. You don't want to sleep through your life. You want to fully live it.

Rewrite Your Inner Dialogue

How do you rewrite your inner dialogue?

1) The first step is to notice your thoughts and become familiar with your negative thoughts, feelings, and sensations. For

example, what goes through your head at that moment. Maybe the headaches that you get so often are the result of stressful thoughts that you have about your weight. Negative thoughts produce negative feelings, which in turn create physical and psychological pain.

2) Identify your talking traps. Pay attention to what you say. The words you use are powerful. They can lead you to see possibilities or impossibilities instead. The moment that you feel that you are tensing up with fear or stress, try to pinpoint the language you use just before you tense up.

3) Transcribe your mental narrative. Think about your goals and see what negative thoughts rise at that moment. Listen to your internal dialogue, visualize yourself going through the motions of accomplishing your goals. What would it be like? As you think about accomplishing your goals, what thoughts come up? Are they negative in nature? Now rewrite your mental narrative. Make it positive. Memorize it and keep on practicing it. For example, if you previously thought, "I can never lose weight, I might as well give up," replace that thought with "I'll never know if I can lose weight if I don't try!"

Judging and rejecting parts of yourself causes pain. It is similar to the pain caused by a physical wound. How do you know that you are judging yourself? One simple rule that you might be using to protect yourself is avoiding anything that might aggravate the pain of self-rejection in any way, such as opening up to others or taking risks in life. To avoid more judgments and self-rejection, you might bury yourself in work, make excuses, or get angry. Stopping the judgments on yourself and healing the wounds of hurt and self-rejection can only be done if you truly believe and feel that change is possible for you. And when that realization becomes clear, you can start.

You can start with your thoughts. Get in touch with your self-talk and create a distinction between your critical voice and your healthy voice. I call this process "refuting the critic." But sometimes the critic overpowers the healthy voice. You need to ask yourself what price you pay for listening to the critic rather than to the critical message itself.

It's important at this point to identify your strengths, the genuine assets you have to stop the critic, and be able to accurately assess yourself. The repetition of your strengths is important, since your self-esteem might have been damaged originally when an authority figure repeatedly attacked your self-worth. It takes a great deal of positive repetitions by a new authority—you—to begin to undo the earlier messages. Remember, your goal is self-acceptance, which is a healthy attitude of acceptance and nonjudgmental thinking toward yourself and others.

A great number of psychologists and researchers emphasize the importance of unconditional self-acceptance. For example, Abraham Maslow (1968) said, "The need for love characterizes every human being that is born... No psychological health is possible unless the essential core is accepted, loved, and respected. As we see, love is important for our survival, and if we did not receive it from others, it's good to provide it ourselves". (p.169)

The psychologist Carl Rogers (1957) postulated that self-acceptance, or unconditioned positive regard, does not depend on one's success but rather on people's evaluations of themselves. He made a distinction between self-acceptance and self-esteem. Self-esteem means that a person values herself because she has behaved intelligently, correctly, and competently, while self- acceptance means that the individual fully and unconditionally accepts herself whether or not she behaves intelligently or correctly and whether or not others approve or respect her.

To be self-accepting does not mean to be without a wish to change. It does mean not being at war with ourselves and not denying the reality of what is true at this moment about ourselves. Being able to accept ourselves refers to an attitude of self-value and self-commitment that derives fundamentally from the fact that "I am alive and living."

Albert Ellis, in his book *The Myth of Self-Esteem* (2005), distinguished conditional self-acceptance where our feelings about our self-worth are dependent on achieving some kind of goal (for example, keeping an ideal weight), and unconditional self-acceptance, when we value ourselves irrespective of whether we achieve our goal. David Burns (2001) argued that unconditional self-acceptance and having a healthy view of oneself are linked to not rating ourselves as worthless or inferior. If we accept ourselves for what we are and see ourselves as possessing intrinsic worth whether or not we achieve our goal, we will be less vulnerable to low self-esteem. If we have unconditional self-acceptance, we may feel happier, lighter, more clear-minded, and less stressed.

Unconditional self-acceptance requires self-kindness and self-compassion. We need to stop the constant self-judgment and understand our failures instead of condemning them. Self-acceptance involves clearly seeing the extent to which we harm ourselves through relentless self-criticism. Self-kindness involves more than merely stopping self-judgment. It also involves actively comforting ourselves. We need to give warmth and sympathy from ourselves to ourselves, so that true healing can occur.

Self-compassion does not try to capture and define the worth or essence of who we are. It's not a label, a thought, or an evaluation. Instead, self-compassion is a way of relating to the mystery of who we are rather than managing our self-image so that it's always perfect. Self-compassion honors the fact that all human beings have both strengths and weaknesses. Rather than getting lost in thoughts of being good or bad, we become mindful of our present experience, realizing that it is ever changing and impermanent.

Our successes and failures come and go. They neither define us nor do they determine our worthiness. They are merely part of the process of being alive. Our minds may try to convince us otherwise, but our hearts know that our true value lies in the core experience of being a conscious being who feels and perceives.

Authentic Self Skill-Building Activity

Exercise V

Sit in a quiet and comfortable place for a few minutes. Close your eyes, relax your body and focus on your breathing for a few minutes. Then open your eyes long enough to read the first statement. Then close your eyes again and focus your attention on the statement by repeating it to yourself three times slowly.

If the statement does not feel right for you, bypass it and return to it later, or change it so it feels right. But keep it all positive. Repeat this exercise for an entire week. Notice each day how you feel as you start feeling more comfortable reading the statements. Below I provide you with a few examples of phrases you could practice to help you get in touch with your authentic self or real self.

I'm not a bad person when I act badly; I just acted badly.

I'm not a good person when I act well; I just acted well.

I can accept myself whether I win or lose.

I am not a fool for acting foolishly.

I have faults that I can work on correcting without blaming myself for having them.

I can talk about my weaknesses and failures without judging myself by them.

I am not stupid for acting stupidly.

I can reprimand my behavior without reprimanding myself.

I can praise my behavior without praising myself.

It may be better to succeed, but success does not make me a better person, nor does failure make me into a stupid person.

Practice these phrases as the need arises. You can add some more phrases to the list that you can relate to and use in your daily life. Keep on reinforcing them with your actions. Repetition and more repetition will help you own them after some time. Remember, you are not born with confidence; you create it throughout your life. All the exercises included in this chapter will help you challenge your core belief that tells you that if you failed at something, or they will help to challenge someone's criticism or rejection of you as a totally hopeless failure.

To counter the tendency to put yourself down when things aren't going so well, ask yourself the following questions: "Does this bad situation (mistake, failure, rejection, criticism) take away my good qualities?" Answer the question honestly. Remember, you're talking to yourself about yourself. Soon you might realize that one single mistake does not define the person that you are today. It only defines one single event from a long list of events in your life.

Your life cannot always be flawless, but self-acceptance will always be there waiting for you. In good times and bad times, whether you are on top of the world or at the bottom, self-acceptance, self-respect and self-compassion will keep you going, helping you move to a better place. It takes hard work to break the self-criticizing habits of a lifetime. But at the end of the day, I'm only asking you to allow life to be as it is and open your heart to yourself. Remember, your personality traits are not static. You, their owner, can change them in the direction that works best for you.

CHAPTER IV

Mental Anim-Morphosis
Reclaim Your Brain Power Through
Exercise, Nutrition, and Self-Acceptance

"Physical fitness is not only one of the most important keys to healthy body; it is the basis of dynamic and creative intellectual activity."

John F. Kennedy

The main focus of this chapter is breaking our aging barriers by learning how to keep our brains active as we age. We would all like to maintain our intellectual acumen as we age, but the big question remains: how do we accomplish this important task? In other words, how do we keep our brains youthful and active at any age, but especially at middle age and beyond?

The most rudimentary answer is "Use it, or lose it." As Henry Ford stated, "Anyone who stops learning is old, whether at twenty or eighty, and anyone who keeps learning stays young." The greatest challenge in life is to keep our mind active and agile by constantly stimulating it with new learning, new discoveries, and a fresh outlook on life. It's completely up to us to keep our brains fit.

Improving our mental functioning at any age is living life like Albert Einstein stated, as if "everything in life is a miracle." This is a throwback to the days when we were children, when we kept our minds alert—filled with spontaneity and curiosity, awake at all times, paying attention to the world around us with fresh eyes, listening to and learning from the world around us. A youthful mind is like a toddler's mind: filled with curiosity, playfulness, and an eagerness to learn. The greatest challenge we have is keeping this momentum going throughout our lives. This can be done by challenging our cognitive functioning.

Psychologists such as Piaget (1963), Vygotsky (1979), and others called this mental challenge "improving our cognition." Cognition is our brain's ability to pay attention, identify, and act. It includes our thoughts, decisions, moods, and actions. According to Piaget, in order to improve our cognition we need to improve its main components: alertness, concentration, learning, memory, problem solving, and creativity. All these can be accomplished by actively engaging our brains through thinking, creating, problem solving, learning, exercising, and proper nutrition. We all posess the ability to nourish our brains at any age.

This chapter provides the reader with the necessary understanding and tools to achieve this goal by examining the basic physiology of the brain, learning how the brain forms memories and stores information, and understanding how proper nutrition, exercise, intellectual curiosity, and mental work affects our brains' functioning.

But before you embark on this journey, you need to ask yourself some simple questions: How do I feel about my brain functioning? Do I believe that it declines as I age? Do I believe that keeping it active will keep it stronger longer? Or do I believe that nothing can be done to avoid the deterioration? Do I buy into the myth that tells me that as I age my brain's functioning slows down?

If you are unsure about the answer to the last question, then reading this book is the first step in the right direction. I will provide you with specific mental and physical activities as well as nutritional plans that will boost your brain's stamina as you progress through middle-life and beyond. If this power is neglected, you will quickly see the effects of age, and your life will be filled with excuses such as, "I'm too old," "I can't remember anything," "My memory is fading," and so on.

Mental Health

Exercise I

This exercise will help you become more intimately attuned to your present mental health.

Do you have trouble remembering names?

Do you feel that your memory is declining?

Do you find it more difficult to concentrate?

Do you rely on too much coffee to keep you alert?

Do you find yourself repeating the same stories to the same people?

Do you often forget where you put things?

Do you lose your train of thought while speaking?

Do you have a problems paying attention to people because your mind is wandering?

Do you have a shorter attention span now than you had before?

Few of us can answer "no" to all these questions regardless of our age. But if your answers are "yes" to most of these questions, it could be that you are suffering from mental fatigue. Most of the time, mental fatigue can be easily corrected by changes in lifestyle, such as diet, exercise, stress reduction, and mental activity. This chapter addresses all of the above minor irritants that might cause you mental fatigue.

The Anatomy of the Mind

Our brain controls every thought, feeling, emotion, personality trait, dream, movement, muscle, and breath that we take. Our body's information system is built from billions of interconnecting cells called neurons, or nerve cells. Our neurons are responsible for all the communication of information throughout our brain. They transfer information by releasing chemicals that jump across synapses, the tiny space between the neuron fibers, from one neuron fiber to another. For example, the sensory neurons carry messages from the body's tissues and sensory organs inward to the brain and spinal cord for processing. The brain and spinal cord then send instructions out to the body's tissue via the motor neurons. Each action triggers the release of chemicals called neurotransmitters. Each neurotransmitter travels a designated path in the brain and has a particular effect on our behavior and emotions.

For example, the neurotransmitter called dopamine influences our movement, learning, attention, and emotions. Dopamine is the chemical which causes feelings of motivation and stimulation. Low levels are associated with low motivation, low energy, poor concentration, and some forms of depression. Our dopamine levels can be increased with physical exercise, proper nutrition, and stimulating activities.

Endorphins are natural opiates released in response to pain. They can be considered our body's own morphine or heroin-like substance. Serotonin is another neurotransmitter that affects our mood, feeling of hunger, and sleep cycle. Low levels of serotonin are linked to depression, anxiety, obsessive thinking, and compulsive behaviors. Neurons that are stimulated and used continue to add new synapses, making new connections, but unstimulated neurons lose connections and die off.

Our brain is divided into two equal halves: the right and left hemispheres. These halves are further subdivided into four parts: frontal, parietal, temporal, and occipital lobes. The left hemisphere's functions are processing our incoming visual, tactile, and other sensations from the right side of the body. The right hemisphere does the same for the left side of our body. The left hemisphere of the brain is important in our language processing while the right hemisphere handles our spatial-visual information and emotions.

For many functions both hemispheres are necessary. For example, the right side of the brain is better at figuring out the meaning of a story, but the left hemisphere is better with decoding grammar and syntax. This means that both sides of the brain have to work together when we read.

Our frontal lobes contain our cortex, which has billions of nerve cells joined together by synaptic connections. Planning, remembering, critical-thinking, and decision making all originate in our frontal lobes. Low activity in this part of our brain is associated with short attention-span, impulsivity, and procrastination.

The cortex is the last part of the brain to develop. The part of the cortex that controls physical motor movement develops first. Then the area that controls complex senses such as vision and hearing develops. Last to develop is the part that controls higher order thinking.

In order to speak, many different areas of the cortex must work together. For example, to answer a question, we must first hear it. This involves the primary auditory cortex. Then, movements controlled by the motor cortex are required to speak and respond. Finally, our cortex is responsible for establishing networks and linking everything together throughout our brain.

In our parietal lobes, we track and receive information. For instance, our ability to navigate in our environment is a function of our parietal lobes. Our occipital lobes are the center of our visual information. Much of what we learn depends on sensory information that reaches our brain from the retina. Our occipital lobes and their connections to other parts of our brain are critical for memories and for learning from visual information sources. Our temporal lobes are critical for memory formation, language function, and the processing of auditory sensations.

Toward the back of the brain resides the cerebellum, a center involved in movement, balance, and coordination. When there are problems in the cerebellum, we tend to struggle with physical coordination and experience trouble learning. The last time you watched a gymnast at the top of her form you were watching the cerebellum operating at its highest level.

The cerebellum is also integral to activities not involving movement, such as when we try to solve a problem or just attempt to remember someone's name. The cerebellum is involved in planning activities that precede movement as well. It coordinates smooth skilled movement from the gesture of a dancer to the everyday action of eating without stabbing ourselves in the nose.

The hippocampus together with the cortex is responsible for our brain power. The hippocampus organizes information so that we can store it in our memory and remember it. Here the explicit memories for facts are processed and fed to other brain regions for storage. New brain cells are also formed in this region of the brain. The hippocampus is responsible for making mental maps which help us remember things such as what time we need to go to work or when our next meeting is. It constantly generates newborn nerve cells even into adulthood. But for these nerve cells to survive, they need to be stimulated.

The strongest stimulus is learning because it provides a biochemical stimulus for forming new contacts, or synapses, with other neurons enabling them to survive. These synapses are connections between neurons. They are the junction between the sending neurons and the cell body of the receiving neurons.

A study by D. Hultsch (1988) suggests that maintaining intellectual activity and learning throughout our lives can protect us against cognitive decline in later years. In a longitudinal study in Canada, Hultsch showed that middle-aged individuals who engage in intellectually stimulating projects and people who engage in every day activities, such as reading a daily newspaper, are less likely to suffer decline in mental functioning later on in life.

Most mental deficiencies involve the cortex and the hippocampus. Keeping them functioning and active is the key to our brain's stamina. In other words, just as we must exercise our body to keep it flexible and agile, so too we must exercise our brain to keep it mentally fit. Many of us fall victim to the fact that life is easier when it's predictable. As a result we tend to ignore new experiences or fail to seek out new learning as we age. We get settled in routines that require little thinking and leave us unchallenged and stuck, which then leads to mental decline.

Our culture instills in us the belief that as we age our brain's power diminishes and nothing can be done about it. However, scientists are making dramatic gains in their understanding of how our brain works, from the biochemistry of synapses to the operations of the important regions of the brain such as the hippocampus, which is involved in memory formation.

Research shows that older people in cultures in which aging adults are held in high esteem, such as China, are less likely to show memory loss than are those living in cultures where there's an expectation that memory will decline. Similarly, when middle-aged people in Western societies are reminded of the advantages of age, such as age bringing wisdom, they tend to do better on tests of memory (Dixon, 2007).

Even when people show declines in memory during later adulthood, these deficits are limited to certain types of memory. For example, losses tend to be limited to episodic memories that relate to specific experiences in people's lives. Other types of memories such as semantic memories, or knowledge of facts, and explicit memories, or memories that we aren't consciously aware of, are not effected by age.

Let's examine what brain functions are involved in everyday tasks. Suppose you decide to buy a newspaper. You need to decide where to buy it. Then you need to walk down the street to the newspaper stand. All this requires the formulation by the brain of a motor program for walking and thereby getting some exercise. Additionally, counting the money and getting the correct change involves regions of our brain. Ten minutes later, you arrive back home with the paper.

Each activity involves different motor programs engaging different muscle groups and different patterns of action. It's the prefrontal lobes that engineer premotor programs. They then dispatch their orders to the motor cortex and the cerebellum, which together carry out the desired action. For example, when we learn something new, we are engaging our brain's primary motor cortex and prefrontal cortex. While the prefrontal cortex is drawing up the plan of action, the motor cortex is practicing it. After we have learned or enhanced our performance, the brain consolidates the memory for what we've learned.

By using our brain every day in challenging activities and problem solving, our brain makes use of its plasticity, which creates new brain cells. By keeping our brain active by thinking, remembering, learning, and creating, we protect our brain against age-associated memory loss.

Most mental decline is not due to the steady death of nerve cells but rather to the thinning out of the number of dendrites, the branches of nerve cells that directly receive and process information from other nerve cells. These branches form the basis of memory. Growing dendrites was only thought to be possible in the brains of children, but more recent research has shown that old neurons can grow dendrites and compensate for losses (Stephen Buell 2002, Science, vol. 206) Discoveries like these are the basis for the new theories of brain exercises. Just as physical training helps maintain physical fitness, brain exercises help maintain mental fitness.

The Five Systems of Memory

Our memories underlie our uniquely human ability to experience our environment and then remember and learn. Our brain receives information, stores it for moments, days, or years, then later recalls it when needed. Memory is the mental process of bringing the past back into the present. Our working memory contains all that we are aware of and working on right now. This form of memory is commonly referred to as our attention span. Information is held here long enough to make a decision, and then either it is lost or sent on to storage for later use. If it's transferred into our storage, it becomes part of our long-term memory.

Working memory, also called short-term memory, is transient in nature, which means that if it's not stored in long-term memory the information will be lost after it is used. Working memory is used for all sorts of things such as planning, questioning, and problem solving. When we want to remember something, our working memory contains a temporary memory of our present experience as well as parts of memories that have been stored as long-term memory. As long as the information is in our working memory, we can think about it and recall the necessary information.

Working memory functions better when it's not overloaded. Paying attention to relevant information is key. Attention deficits have been identified as a primary cause of memory difficulties encountered as we age. It is natural to experience attention problems as we age, but it is something that needs to be actively combated with memory exercises.

The first stage of memory is the sensory component, which allows information to enter the working memory through our senses for encoding. Distractions in attention will impair memory at this stage. For example, if the radio distracts our attention, we're not very likely to retain what our friend is trying to tell us. Therefore, given the changes in attention as we age, it's important to "pay attention to our own attention or inattention."

Long-term memory is where we keep information for later use. It contains the stored, permanent information that we have committed to memory to be retrieved later. Long-term memory is made up of both semantic and episodic memory. Semantic memory includes all the general information that we have gathered in our long-term memories that are not linked by time or place. It involves data related to what, why, or who. Episodic memory is in charge of the information associated with the time and place at which we have learned the information and formed our memory. This memory acts as the memory for when and where. For example, remembering that you spoke to your friend last night is an episodic memory (when). Remembering that your friend lost her valet is a semantic memory (what).

Memory consists of two phases. The first phase is encoding. Once we come in contact with the information to be remembered, our brain develops a code which becomes a record of the experience. This information is taken in from the environment through our senses where it's organized and stored. The second phase is recall or retrieval, which is our ability to recall the information.

The importance of paying attention to detail cannot be overemphasized. If we become preoccupied with other things, it will become increasingly more difficult to remember the things we need for later. What are the things that could infringe upon our memory? To get our brain to function optimally, we need to learn how to diminish the influence of interfering factors such as difficulties in paying attention, difficulties in focus, organizational problems, anxiety, and stress.

Let's take a closer look at what happens when we experience performance anxiety. We become worried, and we cannot think clearly. Negative thoughts start popping up in our mind, exerting a powerful destructive effect on our brain's functioning, resulting in confusion and a strong desire to give up.

Stress is another significant impediment to our memory functioning. Stress can interfere with our concentration and ability to process information. Stress is especially notable as we age because we have accumulated many stressors throughout our years. Some simple coping strategies to reduce stress from our lives include taking control of our lives, getting organized, doing one thing at the time, learning to manage our time well, learning to say no when necessary, exercising, and maintaining a healthy life. When we experience stress, we lack creativity and return to the same old ways, even if they don't work well and cause us to experience inertia, which is when we give up.

Stress has the power to drain our brain acumen and physical strength. For example, a constant noise that we could experience through our stream of thoughts, evaluations, judgments, emotions, agitation, or repeated negative thoughts may cause us to develop an inability to concentrate clearly on the intricacies that we face throughout the day. Reducing these types of mental noises allows us to find more mental clarity with less physical effort and to be more successful in our endeavors.

Learning how to eliminate these types of impediments enhances our brain's power as well as our physical and mental stamina. The brain cannot pay attention to everything at once, but it has the capacity to attend and select what it will attend to. We can increase our attention span by eliminating distractions and training ourselves to pay better attention, by noticing more and paying attention to more details, by setting goals for ourselves and by monitoring our progress.

Improving Your Brain Power

Physical Training

When it comes to our brain, exercise acts like the fountain of youth. It boosts blood flow, increases the brain's use of oxygen, and improves our brain response to stress. Physical brain training exercises stimulate the birth of new neurons and connect them to one another. This strengthens their learning, remembering, and creative abilities and improves the brain's functioning because more oxygen is entering our brain cells. Oxygen is crucial to our optimal brain functioning.

Thirty minutes of walking five to six times a week increases blood flow to our brains, enlarges our frontal lobes, adds new memory-recording neurons in our hippocampus, and replenishes some of the cells lost in the aging process. Moderate aerobics, which make us breathe faster and increase our heart rates, are the most powerful trigger of new cell production in the brain.

According to recent studies, aerobically fit individuals tend to have higher cognitive abilities than sedentary people. They seem to process information more quickly and more easily than their inactive counterparts. Exercise helps normalize brain chemistry and restores mental equilibrium. Studies are pointing to regular physical activity as an alternative to many drugs used for mild depression. And unlike many medications, exercise delivers only positive side effects.

Just thirty minutes of brisk walking four to five times a week dramatically improves brain health, heart functioning, mood, stamina, and brain power. Walking requires moving large muscle in our legs and hips to propel us forward and keep us balanced.

In addition to formal exercises, we can also boost brain functioning by participating in informal physical activities such as gardening, golfing, tennis, cleaning, or playing with children. Remember, it's not about how well we do these activities; it's just about doing them!

Another important exercise that increases our brain's stamina is strength training. Strength training exercises increase our ability to function more efficiently in our day to day living by increasing our muscle mass. Strong muscles allow us to carry heavy grocery bags for a few blocks with little effort or do yard work and household chores with ease. All these activities makes us feel stronger, healthier, and less stressed. When we accomplish different tasks more easily our attitude is more positive and our state of mind is clearer and more productive.

No Equipment Required

Exercise II

The following exercises require no special equipment and can be done at home. These exercises are designed to train the muscles using patterns they have to execute every day. We can use our own body weight to build strength by doing push-ups, squats, and lunges.

Try doing fifteen repetitions with excellent form:

Squats: We do this type of exercise during all sorts of daily activities such as cleaning, gardening, or just taking care of children. Doing multiple squats strengthens muscles in our upper legs, hips, and back. Stand with your feet about shoulder width apart, knees slightly bent, hands resting on your hips. Maintain proper posture, chest up, abs tight with a natural arch in your lower back, and unlocked knees. Lower your hips back behind you and down toward the floor. Push back up to the starting position.

Lunges: These primarily strengthen the muscles in our upper legs and hips. The lunge is another movement we do multiple times a day. We may do a lunge when we reach down to pick something up, when we get down on the floor or up from the floor, when we reach forward or to the side for something, or when we vacuum or do yard work. Stand with your feet hip width apart, one leg in front of the other. Maintain proper body alignment. Keeping your torso upright, bend both knees and lower yourself straight down toward the floor until your back knee is an inch from the floor and your front leg is parallel to the floor. Push back up to the starting position.

Push-ups: Push-ups are great for strengthening our upper body, chest, shoulders, back, and upper arms as well as helping with our balance and stabilizing muscles in our core. We do push-ups when we bend down to pick up something, when we vacuum, when we do gardening, or just picking up our child. Lie on your stomach and place your hands on the floor a few inches to either side of your chest so that your elbows are bent about ninety degrees. Keeping your knees on the floor and your back straight, push your body up until your elbows are straight. Your body should form a straight line from the top of your head to your knees. Keeping your body straight by engaging your abdominal muscle, lower yourself toward the floor until your chest almost touches the floor. Push back up to the starting position.

Repeat these exercises three times. Each time you should include fifteen reps. After you finish, you need to stretch for flexibility and balance. (Stretching exercises will be discussed in the following chapter). No matter how you feel today, a healthier and sharper you is achievable.

Researchers have found that living a sedentary lifestyle constricts our circulation to our muscles and brain. We use fewer pathways in our brains, and with less use our pathways become slow and weak. The results are fading memories and poor coordination. Without a vibrant brain, it's difficult to change our thinking about our own aging. Furthermore, we might have a hard time making the connection between our inactivity and the decline in our memory.

Mental Exercises: Mental Workouts

Exercise III

Review Your Day

This is a memory building exercise that you can practice every evening before you fall asleep. Visually reconstruct everything you have done during the day. Start with the most recent thing you did, and work backwards step-by-step to reconstruct your day. Put in as many small details as you can remember.

Example: I am lying in bed, relaxed and I am thinking of what I did during my day. I walked to my bedroom from the bathroom after taking off my make-up, brushing my teeth, putting night cream on my face and hands. I walked to my bedroom, undressed, put on my night gown, walked to my bed, fixed my pillow, lay down, and started thinking about my day. Before that I made myself a cup of tea in the kitchen...

Go on and on until you get to the morning. Practice this mental exercise for a month, the results will be great.

Write Your Memoirs

This exercise, like the previous one, increases your mental ability and sharpens your mind. Recalling previous events requires a strong memory, which could be improved by using photo albums, letters, or just by taking a walk down memory lane. Write down your life story without including too many details. Rather, write it as a sequence of dramatic, uplifting, momentous, and relevant scenes. Challenge your brain and try to remember the events in the order in which they happened.

Go Shopping Without a List

Make a shopping list at home before going out shopping. Leave the list at home and try to remember the items that were on the list. When you return home, look at the list and see how many things you forgot to get. Do this for a few weeks and challenge yourself to remember more every week. Also introduce the idea of no more one-stop shopping. For example, explore an old-fashioned hardware store as opposed to a super-store, or explore a flea market or a small bookstore that might offer more opportunities for genuine social interactions with other people. You are more likely to encounter recommendations from the staff related to your interests, as well as develop new interests, in a novel environment more conducive to thinking and learning.

Be as Receptive as a Baby

As we grow up, our brain undergoes a pruning process that narrows our perception of life and can lead to limited creativity and decreased ability to problem solve. This pruning also limits our ability to "be in the now" and leaves us less open and less flexible. A baby's brain, on the other hand, has an amazing ability to sort through lots of excess information and remain receptive to discovering highly rewarding solutions and innovative concepts. A baby's brain notices the beauty around it and lives very much in the "now." You could recapture a baby's state of mind if you consciously choose to live mindfully, in the now, looking at new experiences with fresh eyes, learning to reduce your inhibitors, and observe without judgment or criticism. Learn as a baby does through your five senses. Listen to beautiful music or to the sounds of nature. Feel the texture of things. Look at your world with fresh eyes. Taste things as if for the first time.

Play and Games

It has been scientifically proven that play and games sharpen children's minds, which leads to more brain power. Piaget (1965), one of the leading psychologists of our time, studied cognitive development throughout adulthood and proved that "our brain power is enhanced by active thinking. If we stop thinking and we operate as robots, our mental ability will deteriorate regardless of our age. One the other hand, if we sustain active brain functioning, then our brain power will be sustained and strengthened regardless of our age. Piaget's basic philosophy was "if we don't use it, we lose it," and this could happen at any age.

Piaget also argued that some of us never develop our highest mental ability, which he calls "formal operational thinking." This type of thinking includes flexibility, creativity, inquiry, exploring new possibilities, hypothetical and logical thinking and reasoning as well as awareness of our own thinking, which he called "metacognition." We can achieve this higher order thinking at any age during our life time, but we need to be ready to believe that it is possible. So changing and challenging our belief to grow wiser and stronger each day is within our reach. We just need to reach out and grab it. Let's continue playing, creating, and imagining the way we did in our early childhood years.

Walking Mindfully

While you are out for a walk, make mental notes of each storefront. Notice window displays and any sounds you hear and can associate with each store. Pay attention to smells from foods and any other clues that will trigger your memory. After you complete your walk, write down the names of the stores in order. Then write down what was featured in their respective windows. If you cannot recall all the stores, repeat the same walk the next day and do the same. When you get home, recreate your walk and see how many more details you remembered. By doing this exercise you are building a personal palace of memories.

Get in the Play

Play any games such as crossword puzzles, chess, board games, or any other game that makes you think. All these will boost your memory as well as sharpen your visual and spatial skills. The following are a list of brain-boosting activities that also involve play:

- Reading.
- Watching intellectually stimulating shows instead of programs for entertainment.
- Choosing hobbies that stimulate different parts of your brain.
- Learning something new, like a new language.
- Learning to play chess to weigh dozens of possible moves and stimulate visual-spatial thinking.
- Developing your computer skills to improve your working-memory capacity.
- Designing, planning, and building a home project such as a kitchen, office, or garden.

Take an Alternative Route to Work

Break your routine. This is especially good if you are into routines or habits. You can increase your brain power if you change your daily routines by introducing new ideas to your old existing habits.

Mental practice is to the mind what physical exercise is to your body and mind. Don't ask yourself how smart you are, but rather how you are smart. Don't stop challenging your brain on a daily basis. Be a perpetual student for life, i.e. a lifelong learner. For example, you can take continuing education courses, or you can learn a new language or be a gourmet cook. The world around you has endless and fascinating new experiences just waiting for you to explore.

Make exercise a habit, whether physical or mental. A habit is a series of actions your brain executes when you tell it to do so. But it takes time and many repetitions before your brain learns to perform a function automatically. The best chance of making exercise a habit is to schedule a specific time and place to exercise every day. It's important to vary the routine to prevent boredom and keep you motivated. After a few weeks of sticking to the routine, you no longer think about whether or not to be physically and mentally active. You do it automatically.

Nutrition for Your Brain

Nutrition, perhaps more than any other factor, plays an essential role in our overall health, including brain functioning. The reason for this is simple: the food we eat affects virtually every cell, organ, and system in our bodies. Healthy food provides our cells with everything they need to function well, reproduce, and repair damage from a variety of sources.

The brain is the most demanding organ in our body when it comes to energy requirements. The brain's primary fuel is glucose or simple sugar, essential fats (such as omega-3 and omega-6 fatty acids), amino acids, vitamins (E, C, B12), and the antioxidants contained in fruits and vegetables.

Glucose provides energy for the hippocampus and provides energy to all other working parts of the brain. The source of glucose is simple sugars, fruits, vegetables, and grains.

Amino acids are the major building blocks for proteins. They can be obtained from meats, fish, and dairy products. Essential fats, such as omega-3 and omega-6 are found in fatty fish, nuts, avocados, legumes, and vegetable oils.

But the big question that looms before us is what keeps us from achieving good eating habits? And where do we get the willpower to do so? As I discussed earlier in this chapter, there are three neurotransmitters that determine how much control we have over ourselves and how well are we able to stick to eating well. Dopamine serves as a drive chemical in our brain; serotonin as a happy, flexible chemical; and endorphins serve as the brain's natural pleasure and painkilling chemical.

The strength and weakness of each of these neurotransmitters determines how much control we have over ourselves. When these chemicals are balanced in our brain, we can be focus and have control our cravings. But when these chemicals are off balance, we often get off track and can no longer focus on our goals. Regaining our brain's balance can be done simply by maintaining a healthy blood sugar level, by eating smaller meals more frequently, and by creating specific goals for ourselves.

Healthy Foods

Fruits: All fresh and frozen fruits.

Vegetables: Most fresh, frozen, or canned vegetables without sugar or oil as well as potatoes: white, red and sweet.

Whole grains: Brown and wild rice, hot cereals cooked without added sugar, dried fruits or nuts, cream of rice, one-hundred percent bran, cream of wheat, oatmeal, pasta, whole wheat, whole grain ready to eat cereals without added sugar, barley, polenta, quinoa, and whole wheat couscous.

Fruits and vegetables are what we call brain foods. Fruits contain antioxidants, which protect our bodies and brains from toxicities. Antioxidants nourish and defend our body's cells, including our neurons, against the damages of oxidative stress, as well as help prevent the buildup of plaque in our arteries and ensure strong blood flow to our brains. Vegetables, such as leafy greens (spinach, broccoli, kale, cauliflower, cabbage, and Brussels sprouts), were found to help improve our memory and prevent memory loss.

Non-fat dairy: Fat free cheeses, fat free milk, fat free yogurt, fat free sour cream, fat free soy cheese, soy milk, and soy yogurt are all healthy options.

Lean proteins: Beef, chicken, lamb, pork, turkey, and veal can be quite healthy when trimmed of fat with all skin removed. Dried beans, dried peas, eggs, lentils, tofu, vegetarian burgers, and nuts are also good sources of protein. Protein increases brain functioning. Start with a high protein breakfast, and keep the carbohydrates low.

Dietary fats are important components of the outer wall of the brain cells and allow easy transmission of signals back and forth from the brain to the far parts of our body. Our brain is approximately two-thirds fat. We need to distinguish between good fats and bad fats. Bad fats (saturated fats) are associated with the hardening of our arteries and plaque formation, which accumulates in the blood vessels and blocks the free flow of blood to the heart and brain. Saturated fats are found in red meats, egg yolks, and dairy foods like butter and whole milk.

Essential good fats (unsaturated fats): These include omega-3 and omega-6 fatty acids. Foods rich in omega-3 fatty acids include salmon, sardines, herring, tuna, mackerel, trout, walnuts and walnut oil, flaxseed, flaxseed oil, canola oil, olive oil, nuts, and avocado.

Making these foods a regular part of our daily nutrition is vital for maintaining optimal brain functioning. Foods rich in omega-6 fatty acids include nuts, legumes, and most vegetable oils. Eating these in moderation is important. Avoid eating more than a serving once or twice a week of high fat red meats, dairy products, or many processed foods as these contain saturated fats that are harmful to our brain.

Water: Water is essential for our brain and body's functioning. We need to include in our daily routine at least eight large glasses of water to stay hydrated and healthy.

Food to Stay Away From

What our brain does not need are food high in salt, processed foods high in sugar, or foods high in saturated fats or high in trans fats.

The following should be eliminated from your diet: white flour, white rice, white sugar, white potatoes, or white pasta. Avoid sugar foods such as candies, cookies, and cakes because they increase adrenaline in the blood level, which in turn hinders your concentration, increases anxiety and hyperactivity, and slows down your ability to concentrate. Also eliminate more than two cups of coffee per day and switch to green tea or water. Tea has strong antioxidant properties.

Final Recommendations

To get started, watch your calorie intake, drink plenty of water, increase good fats and decrease bad fats. Increase good carbs and decrease bad carbs, eliminate artificial sweeteners, and reduce salt intake. Plan to have regular snacks and regular meals. Add herbs and spices to boost your food. Sit down when you eat, eat slowly, and watch your portion size. Don't talk while chewing your food, so all your senses are turn inward and you can enjoy the taste and smell of your food. Include a diet rich in vegetables, fruits, fish, olive oil, nuts, whole grains, and legumes. Finally, include fiber in your daily meals.

Our brain plasticity is maintained throughout our life span, given the right challenge. For example, if we engage in the same tasks day in and day out, our brain is stimulated less and its plasticity deteriorates. It's important to embrace new opportunities to optimize our brain's functioning. Optimal brain functioning involves new activities, new skills, and new challenges. The danger that we face in doing the same things every day is that our brains become unchallenged, resulting in mental decline and we will buy into the mind-set that with age our mental energy diminishes. As a result, we no longer can engage in mind-challenging activities, such as taking a class, or learning a new skill, picking up a new hobby, and so on. Learning new skills stimulates our functioning and keeps the brain agile longer.

The frequency and variety of brain activities, whether physical or mental, is the key to our health. Remember, every form of movement stimulates the brain, and every new thought affects our body. This mind-body connection is important, and mind-body exercises combine awareness and mental focus. With body movement and controlled breathing we can enhance both our physical and mental well-being.

No more jokes about "senior moments." Keeping your brain sharp is easier than you think. Start by stimulating your mind with mental exercises. Look at what you are currently doing for mental stimulation. If it's watching reality shows and reading only tabloid magazines, you are in real trouble. You need to stretch your brain, continue learning, and expose yourself to new learning experiences. It could be as simple as completing a crossword puzzle or as complex as learning a new language.

Now, take a look at your eating habits and your daily activity level. Do you walk at least thirty minutes a day? Do you eat properly? What are your eating habits? Remember all of these factors together are what keep your brain and your body healthy. By following these simple exercises and tips you will realize that aging is not a disease to be avoided at any cost, but rather a journey of personal growth.

CHAPTER V

Physical Anim-Morphosis through Fitness and Exercise

"Lack of activity destroys the good condition of human being, while movement and physical exercise saves it and preserves it."

Plato, 370 B.C.

"Motion is a good thing for both soul and body, and immobility is bad."

Socrates, 153 B.C.

"Our body is a machine for living."

Leo Tolstoy, (1828 – 1910)

Daily, we are inundated from every source possible (books, TV, magazines, doctors, billboards, journals and so on) about the benefits that physical exercise has on our body and mind and the health hazards a sedentary lifestyle brings. So how come not everyone is exercising or keeping active in some way?

This chapter gives you the tools to rewrite your own individual lifestyle by understanding the relationship between physical fitness and mental wellness, by identifying your self-sabotaging patterns of behavior, and by helping you maintain control over how and when you exercise. I am in no way claiming that physical exercise wipes away all your problems, but rather that when you begin to take care of yourself physically, you develop stamina for managing the complexities of life.

Many of us become sedentary as we get older without realizing it. Life slows down when the kids move out and we start having fewer obligations. We may take time to read more, watch TV, sit and talk on the phone, and so on. We also tend to do less recreational activities. We might even cut down on work around the house. Meanwhile, our bodies are adapting; our muscles become stiffer. We get weaker since our muscles do not support our joints as well, and slowly we become what we do or don't do.

The question is "Are you ready to learn how to love and respect your body so that it works for you and not against you?" And if your answer is "yes," then reading this chapter is the first step in the right direction since creating an individualized healthy lifestyle with proper fitness and nutrition is the main focus of the next two chapters.

For me, working out has helped me manage my stress, given me vitality, and helped me deal more clearly with my emotions. After working out, my head is clearer, and I feel more in control of things in my life. Through proper nutrition and physical activity, I have gained a great deal of self-confidence. Confidence was the essential ingredient I needed to let go of old behaviors that no longer worked for me. I revamped and reconditioned my lifestyle which gave me a strong sense of self-empowerment.

If you are reading this book, I'm assuming that there are certain things you would like to change about yourself, including your body. For example, you might want to tighten your stomach muscles, strengthen your body's stamina, improve your posture, or reduce your stress level without having to take medicine. This chapter will help you get started.

It is important for us to acknowledge that our bodies are designed to move throughout our lifetime. Our ability to feel strong and capable in our bodies develops early in our lives. As a child, the essential element to feel safe and secure in the world comes from our body. Exercise and breathing fresh air are as essential to our body as food and water.

Our bodies help us to build a sense of mastery over our world. What we today call total physical fitness (strength, endurance, and flexibility) we naturally developed as children through play and different types of activities. As we become older and life becomes more complex, many times we get distracted and become disconnected from our body's most essential need: movement. Movement needs to be part of our daily commitment to ourselves and our wellbeing.

We all know that there is an immutable biology of aging: our hair gets gray, gravity takes its toll, and movies and buses go to half price. Our maximum heart rate declines regardless of how active we are, and we also look older no matter what. Our arteries lose some of their elasticity and they become stiff over time. Our brain arteries stiffen, reducing blood flow, and our metabolism changes. Our eyesight weakens, and we might need glasses. But we can change many of these things by changing some of our behaviors and beliefs. For example, we can change and have more control over our aches and pains or over our anxiety, depression, or stress level by simply paying more attention to our body's cues and taking proper care of them. Overriding those default signals and changing our lifestyle by embracing growth instead of decay is all within our power. The key to accomplishing all these things is daily exercise, healthy nutrition, emotional commitment to a healthy lifestyle, and a real engagement with living. Aging is up to nature, but decay is up to us.

An easy message to internalize at this point is everything we eat, everything we do physically, everything we think and feel, and every emotion we experience changes our body and brain physically. Researchers have found that physical activity and active involvement in daily life trigger great waves of growth. Our bones strengthen and joint health increases. Our heart and circulatory functions increase to supply the blood and oxygen to our muscles. Our muscles become stronger and more coordinated. Our joints get lubricated, decreasing our chances of developing arthritis or other joint conditions. Our good cholesterol (HDL) increases. Our immune function increases to repair the ongoing wear and tear of minor infections, cuts, and bruises. Our brain gets stimulated and our stress level decreases to ignite the spark of life. Activity increases our energy level, motivation, and self-esteem. We feel better about ourselves, have more fun, and improve our overall quality of life.

With this in mind, think of the messages that your brain is getting from the way you live today, and think about whether it tells your body to grow or decay. The big question that this chapter addresses is "How do you choose between decay and growth, between older and younger?"

First, we need to develop a caring and respectful attitude toward our body. This type of attitude tends to positively influence our feelings toward our core self. Our body could be considered as a metaphor for our core self, which simply means that the way we experience our bodies is similar to the way we experience our core self. For example, you might say to yourself, "I would appreciate my body more if it didn't have so many wrinkles." What you are doing is placing harsh conditions on loving your core self. If you are hard on your physical imperfections, it's easier to experience your core self in a similar way. In other words, if you don't like the way you look, then you don't like yourself.

Second, we need to honestly examine the barriers standing in the way of embracing a healthy lifestyle and understand why, even though we are interested in starting to increase our level of activity, something is holding us back. We might come up with good reasons why we cannot be more active or change our lifestyle. Breaking through some of our resistance is key to advancing on our road toward physical anim-morphosis, or self-change.

One frequently used reason for inactivity is time. We often tell ourselves, "I just can't find the time." Sometimes we just need a little bit of creativity to find thirty minutes or so on most days in order to meet the weekly recommendation. Creativity could include putting the stationary bike in front of the T.V. Another frequently used reason for inactivity is exhaustion: "I'm so tired, I have no energy." But by gradually increasing our activity level, we will actually gain energy. Or you may think to yourself, "Exercising is so boring and redundant." But exercise can be fun if we use a variety of exercises, discover new and different ways of increasing our physical stamina, and enlist the people we love so that we have a support system. An important rule of thumb is to develop self-awareness, knowledge, curiosity, a sense of commitment, and to realize what the benefits of keeping active are in our lives. It is up to us to find a good reason to change our lifestyle.

Third, we need to set up an exercise routine that works for us. We need to set aside a daily time just for ourselves and no one else. It's important to get into the routine of working out without any interruptions.

When we think about exercise that will prolong our lives and health, our goal should be to find vigorous, demanding physical activity. Vigorous exercise creates lactic acid, which can greatly benefit the heart as well as remove toxic metals that accumulate in our bodies. Many researchers and gerontologists have found that exercise is the closest thing to an anti-aging pill that exists today.

Form a Positive Attitude

When choosing an exercise, it's important to choose one that you will actually do. Women can find joy and fitness in a wide variety of activities ranging from walking, bike riding, dancing, jogging, aerobics, using the treadmill, skiing, and playing tennis to any other outdoor activities such as gardening, cleaning the yard, and snow plowing.

Make a strong commitment to move your body. Committing to some form of activity five to six times a week for thirty minutes is imperative. Commit yourself to an exercise program for at least one month. By then your body will crave the exercise routine, and you will not be able to stop and go back to your sedentary lifestyle.

Learn proper breathing through your nose. Once you train your body to use oxygen efficiently, you will find that you can, for example, walk faster with less effort and feel more energized.

Get in touch with the self-sabotaging behaviors that you may have acquired throughout the years. Start slowly: do less in the beginning than you are capable of. Your body will react positively because the message you are sending is that you know how to take care of it and not push it to exhaustion.

Don't get discouraged, and remember that although your strength and stamina is a gradual process, most of us experience fitness as a series of quantum leaps. One day you can barely drag yourself around the block while the next day walking for sixty minutes seems so easy and natural. You'll soon find that regular, appropriate exercise will help you create a sense of power and well-being that is well worth any difficulties you might experience from time to time.

Listen to your body. The more you pay attention to how you feel during a workout (and after), the more accustomed you will become to deciding how hard to push yourself. When you become comfortable with your routine, it is time to add more repetitions, more weight, or longer or harder cardio—whether it's straight walking, running, working on a treadmill or any other machine—so you could see more visible results in your body.

Exercise for Life

A combination of some kind of aerobic and resistance activities are best for our cardiovascular muscles and metabolic systems. This means that we need to do several resistance exercises for the upper and lower body a few times a week and about thirty minutes of aerobic activity (e.g. walking, cycling, swimming, or sports) on most days of the week.

Remember, fitness involves proper breathing, flexibility, and alignment. The effects of life's complexities wear us down, resulting in muscle, flexibility, and alignment deterioration over time unless we do something about it. For example, yoga, Pilates, and stretching exercises are great ways to relax, stretch, and maintain our body in proper alignment.

A complete fitness program includes exercises to enhance flexibility, strength, and endurance. Strength training, like weight lifting, slows muscular atrophy, the process by which muscles shrink. Lifting weights increases our lean body mass, since that mass decreases as we get older. The more lean muscle we have, the higher our resting metabolic rate, and the more calories we burn each day while doing nothing. Resistance training increases bone density, which in later life helps avoid osteoporosis. More muscle means that our metabolic rate will be higher, so we will burn more calories. Resistance work is important for maintaining strong bones and healthy joints as the muscles supporting those joints strengthen and provide us with more support.

Endurance training strengthens our heart and facilitates the transportation of oxygen cells throughout our bodies. It also helps reduce our fat levels by converting fat into fuel for exercise. Cardiovascular exercise can help us feel refreshed and alert, and it is associated with improved memory and learning. It has long been known that cardiovascular exercise reduces stress by keeping our fat levels down as well as reducing bad cholesterol in our arteries.

Flexibility exercises are important because with age our flexibility tends to decline. Stretching keeps our tendons and muscles flexible and helps joints and muscles maintain a full range of motion. It also feels good and can have a soothing effect.

Improving muscle tone through weight-bearing exercises can improve our posture and reduce back pain. Muscles respond well to regular activity, which means that we can benefit by systematically exercising the major muscle groups in our arms, legs, and trunk.

There are nine major muscle groups in our bodies: chest, back, shoulders, biceps, triceps, quadriceps, hamstrings, glutes, calves, and abdominals.

In the beginning of any exercise routine, it's important to train your large muscle group and work towards the smaller ones. Start with the muscles of the torso (chest, back, and shoulders), then your arms (biceps and triceps), followed by the muscles of the quadriceps, hamstrings and abdominals. When training your upper body, it's best to alternate between pushing and pulling movements. The chest, shoulders and triceps are used to push a weight, while the back and biceps are pulling mechanisms. It's important to use different exercises for each muscle group and alternate between them, so your body can recover. Recovery is an important component of any exercise program.

Whichever exercises you choose, there are some basics facts that remain the same in any complete fitness program: flexibility, strength, and endurance training.

Get Into the Habit

Exercise habits and routines lead to success. Your body will eventually crave the release of "feel good" chemicals that are released by the neurotransmitters during exercise. Whether the exercise is long or short is less important than the frequency of it. So experiment with a variety of different exercises at the gym, at home, or outdoors. The whole point is to give your body and brain the signals to keep them healthy and functioning well. What is most important is that you are moving in the right direction.

For me, exercise has become an important part of my life. It energizes me, strengthens my body, and gives me a high that lasts for the entire day. I prefer to do my exercise routine in the morning before my life gets filled with daily routines. I feel good, and my body craves the feeling of the good chemicals that are released during my workout.

Getting Started

Start by simply following a few basic facts. Pick a time of the day to exercise, but don't exercise within forty-five minutes of eating. Many of us find it convenient to exercise right before breakfast, lunch, or dinner. Since it is ideal to exercise every day, find a variety of exercises that you can rotate through. It's also a good idea to have some inexpensive pieces of equipment at home. What is most important is that you develop a program that you enjoy and look forward to.

Warm Up

It's very important to warm up before any physical activity in order to lessen the chances of pulling a muscle or ligament. Never over-exert yourself during the warm up since it can cause fatigue by building up your oxygen debt. If you have been inactive for a long time, I recommend beginning with just light daily stretching exercises to help you regain functional range of motion in certain joints and to avoid risk of injury. The most important targets of stretching are the hamstrings, lower back, shins, calves, and quadriceps. Warm-up exercises prepare your body and remove stiffness. In the beginning, exert yourself in each pose to the point where you feel the stretch. Over time you will notice increased strength and flexibility.

Lie on your back and lengthen the spine. Keep the head and neck long. Bring your knees up to your chest, clasp your hands over your knees, and begin to roll slowly from side to side. Breath normally.

Begin by kneeling and sitting with your buttocks on your heels. Lengthen the spine and slightly lift your chest. Look straight ahead and breathe easily. As you inhale, lift your buttocks off your heels and come up to a kneeling position. Relax your shoulders. Then, slowly lower your body, and sit back on your heels. Repeat this exercises ten times with slow movements.

Sit down and extend your legs out in front of you. Stretch through the back of your legs. Than bend your left knees and place the sole of your left foot against the inside of your right thigh. Inhale and lift your arms straight up to the ceiling, and then slowly bend your body forward and down, elongating your spine. Hold this pose for a few seconds, and then slowly come up opening your chest forward. Repeat the same exercises with your other foot.

To begin the cobra pose, lie face down on your stomach. Bring your feet together and hands directly under your shoulders. Then lift your chest forward and up as you press down with your hands. Hold for twenty seconds, than exhale and come down slowly. Next, raise both legs away from the floor. Keep lengthening your entire spine as your legs extend toward your back. Hold for twenty seconds, and then slowly lower your legs.

Sit with your legs extended in front of you. Sit straight with your spine lengthened. Bend your left knee, and bring your heel toward the buttocks just above the inner part of the right knee. Extend your right leg straight in front of you. Now, bring your left hand on to the floor behind you and your right arm on the side of the left knee. As you twist, keep opening your chest to the left and let your head follow the movement. Hold the pose for twenty seconds, and then release slowly. Repeat the same pose on the other side.

Stand straight and bring your arms up toward the ceiling. Slowly bend your body forward and down. Let your knees soften and bring your arms to the floor. Hold the pose for twenty seconds, then come back slowly to your starting position.

Aerobics or Cardio for Endurance

This could include walking, jogging, biking, swimming, aerobics classes, tennis, gardening, spinning, or any other outdoor activity or sport. Start with an exercise that is aerobic in nature, one that requires a high use of oxygen. Set aside thirty minutes five to six days a week. This is your "me time," the time each day that you give to yourself.

Cardio fitness is an important part of getting in shape and improving your overall health. Any exercise that is aerobic—any exercise in which you increase the amount of oxygen you take in and which causes your heart to pump more blood—improves your cardiovascular health and general level of fitness. After a while, you may want to increase the duration of your cardio workout from thirty minutes to forty minutes or increase your frequency to six days a week. Play around with your routine, but don't stop doing it.

The main goal is to get your body moving daily, establish a routine, and set aside time in your weekly schedule to exercise. Remember to give yourself a break when you need it. Listen to your body and acknowledge your progress by rewarding yourself from time to time. This is your "me time," the time you have set aside for yourself and no one else. The more regularly you allow for this time, the more you will discover that you can't do without it. Again, if you are new to exercising or find it difficult to stick to any form of aerobics, the best place to start is walking.

Walking is the perfect initial step for the beginning exerciser because it can eventually lead to other, higher endurance exercises. Do not underestimate the benefits of walking, as very fast walking can actually be more beneficial aerobically than jogging or slow running at the same speed. Walk to your favorite music. Walk with a friend. Walk whenever you can. Practice moderation. If you can't walk one day, don't push yourself. Practice positive thinking during your walks. Use your walking time as personal time for yourself.

Think how good you feel when you exercise, and think about how much stronger you are getting mentally and physically.

Running offers amazing health benefits, and it makes your whole body stronger. You can begin with a quarter mile every two days and slowly build up to one mile twice a week. The benefits of running are innumerable. It improves respiration and circulation. It improves muscle strength and endurance. It improves joint flexibility, balance, and movement. It also increases production of endorphins and improves cognition. Start out with a slow jog for a short duration and distance, and watch it build to running that feels good for you.

Biking comes in many varieties: biking outdoors, biking indoors on a stationary bike, and spinning, which is a popular fitness trend and a great cardio exercise. Here is an example of stationary bicycle workout: three minutes with resistance at eight; one minute with resistance at nine; one minute with resistance at ten; one minute at nine; one minute at eight. Repeat this cycle five to ten times.

Swimming is an excellent aerobic exercise with the big advantage that it is easier to move your limbs in the water because of significant reduction in your apparent weight. That's why swimming and water aerobics are ideal forms of exercises for those who suffer from muscle or joint injury and cannot continue their usual workout routines.

Treadmill workouts are nice because you can alter them gradually to fit your fitness goals. Start with a brisk walk. When ready, proceed to a light jog for two to three minutes (at 5.0-5.5 mph). Increase the incline to 1.0 and continue jogging for two to three minutes. Bring the incline to 3.0 and continue for two to three minutes. Repeat this cycle five to ten times.

Burst training cardio exercises, known as interval training, burn fat and calories faster than continuous intense activity. For example, walk at a fast pace, and then jog for two minutes. Repeat this interval throughout your exercise. Here is an example of a heart pumping thirty-minute workout with interval training: four minutes of fast walking followed by a one-minute run or walking as fast as you can. Continue this training for thirty minutes and then take four minutes to cool down and stretch.

Resistance Training for Strength

When you are doing strength training, you place stress on your muscles and bones, which respond by becoming stronger and leaner. One of the fastest ways to increase muscle mass is by working with resistance weights. First, you need to evaluate your present body strength to know what your endurance range is. If, for example, you lift weights that are too heavy, you could overstress your muscles, ligaments, or tendons. On the other hand, if you lift weights that are too light, your results will be very slow to appear. For safe but quick body sculpting results, you should be performing exercises made up of a fixed number of repetitions. Start with a set of ten, and then slowly try to build it up.

Weight training is one of those activities where you need to pay attention to keep it challenging. The specific number of pounds that you lift is not important. You get stronger over time. What's important is that you are able to execute your exercises in a slow and controlled manner with good posture. This is how you improve your strength. When you do it properly, you should be able to lower the weight and lift it with control. Fast movements mean you're not maximizing your training benefits. Remember: move with control. Execute your exercises smoothly through a full range of motion. Over time, you'll notice a huge difference in your body awareness and ability to control the movement.

Strength training works because it places stress on your muscles. This causes microscopic injury to your muscle cells. During your rest period, your cells repair this damage. That's why it's important to change your routine daily so your muscle cells can repair themselves. Through repair, your muscles become stronger, and you gain more power, strength, and a better control over your body.

The increase in lean muscle mass that results from strength training is key to overall strength and to your body's ability to burn calories. This is because muscle cells require more energy, and also burn more calories, than fat cells. Overall fitness requires a good balance between cardiovascular fitness, endurance, strength, and flexibility.

An important caveat is that muscles need at least forty-eight hours between training sessions to recover and repair. If you are training your entire body daily, your muscles will not have time to build new tissue, and your workout will not be as beneficial. Try to train different muscle groups every second day for optimal benefits.

Chest Sculpting Exercises

Exercise I

Incline Dumbbell Press

Lie face up on an incline bench. Grasp two dumbbells and with your palms facing away from your body, bring them to shoulder level so that they rest just above your armpits. Then press both dumbbells at the same time directly over your chest, moving them toward each other. Feel a contraction in your chest muscles, and then slowly return to the start position. (Three sets of ten reps)

High Cable Crossover

Grasp the two overhead pulley handles. Stand with your feet shoulder width apart. Slowly pull both handles down and across your body in a semicircular movement. Bring your hands together and squeeze your chest muscles so you feel a contraction in the chest area. Then slowly go back to your starting position. (Three sets of ten reps)

Low Cable Crossover

This variation targets the upper chest fibers. Stand with your feet shoulder width apart. Slowly pull both handles up and across the body, creating a semicircular movement. Bring your hands together and squeeze your chest muscles so you feel the contraction in your chest area. Then slowly release, and go back to the start position. (Three sets of ten reps)

Back Muscle Exercises

Exercise II

Front Lat Pull-Down

Grasp the straight bar attached to the pull-down machine with both hands, and secure your knees under the restraint pad. Fully straighten your arms and then slowly pull the bar to your upper chest. Squeeze your shoulders and return to the start position. (Three sets of ten reps)

Seated Row

Sit down in front of the pulley with your feet against the footplate. Keep your knees slightly bent. Pull the V-bar to your lower abdomen. Squeeze your shoulder blades together and then return to the start position. (Three sets of ten reps)

Straight Arm Pull-Down

Grab on to the straight bar attached to a high pulley with both hands. Keep your upper body tilted forward, and slowly pull the bar down until it touches your upper thighs. Release and return to your start position. (Three sets of ten reps)

One Arm Dumbbell Row

Put your right foot firmly on the floor, and place your left hand and left knee on a flat bench. Grasp a dumbbell in your right hand, and let it hang by your side. Keeping your elbow close to your

your body, pull the dumbbell up and back until it touches your hip. Keep your back flat and tight. Then slowly return to the start position. (Three sets of ten reps)

Shoulder Exercises

Exercise III

Front Dumbbell Raise

Grab two dumbbells and allow them to hang by your hips. Slowly raise the dumbbells in front of your body to shoulder level. Then slowly return to the start position. (Three sets of ten reps)

Dumbbell Shoulder Press

Bring two dumbbells to your shoulder level with your palms facing away from your body. Slowly press the dumbbells directly upward and in. Make sure that they touch over your head. Then go back to the start position. (Three sets of ten reps)

Dumbbell Lateral Raise

Grab two dumbbells and allow them to hang by your hips. With your elbows slightly bent, raise the dumbbells up and out to the side of your body. Then return back to the start position. (Three sets of ten reps)

Bicep Exercises

Exercise IV

Bicep Curl

You can do this sitting down or in a standing position. Find an object that weights five pounds to start. You can purchase a small dumbbell or use a container of unopened water or milk. Sit down in a chair, and with your back supported do ten repetitions. With one hand resting on your thigh, slowly extend your elbow on the hand holding the dumbbell and then fully flex your arm. Inhale while flexing your arms and exhale while extending. After completing a round of ten reps, rest half a minute and then repeat. Do this three times with each arm. This exercise strengthens your bicep muscles.

Cable Curl

Grasp a straight bar attached to a low pulley. Slightly bend your knees and press your elbows to your side, keeping them stable throughout the movement. Slowly curl the bar toward your shoulders and contract your biceps. Return to the start position. (Three sets of ten reps)

One Arm Dumbbell Curl

Grasp a dumbbell with your right hand, and place the upper portion of your right arm on an inclined bench. Keeping your upper arm pressed to the bench, slowly curl the dumbbell upward toward your shoulder. Contract your biceps and return to the starting position. Do the same exercise with your left hand as well. (Three sets of ten reps)

Two Arm Dumbbell Curl

You can do the previous exercise using two arms by grabbing a straight bar. (Three sets of ten reps)

Tricep Exercises

Exercise V

Two Handed Tricep Extensions

Grasp a dumbbell with both hands. Raise your arm, bend your elbows, and allow the weight to hang down behind your head. Slowly straighten your arms toward the ceiling. Then slowly lower the weights to the start position. (Three sets of ten reps)

Overhead Rope Extension

Turn your back toward the cable pulley. Bend forward and with both arms grasp the ropes attached to the pulley. Then slowly straighten your arms, keeping your elbows back. Contract your triceps. Return to the starting position. (Three sets of ten reps)

Tricep Press-Down

Grasp a straight bar attached to a high pulley machine. With your knees slightly bent, bend your arms so that your elbows form a ninety-degree angle. Keep your elbows in at your sides. Slowly straighten your arms. Contract your triceps and then return to the start position. (Three sets of ten reps)

Tricep Dip

Begin by placing your heels on the floor and your hands at the end of a flat bench, keeping your arms straight. Slowly, bend your elbows allowing your butt to go down bellow the level of the bench. Then straighten your arms to return to the start position. (Three sets of ten reps)

Tricep Extension

Stand with your feet hip-width apart. Take a dumbbell in one hand and lift your arm towards the ceiling. Then bend your elbow to drop the arm down behind your shoulder. Support your elbow with your other hand, and keep your upper body straight. Next, move your arm back to your initial position by extending the bent arm upwards and pressing the weight toward the ceiling. Then lower your arm. Repeat this movement slowly ten times. Do the same movement with your other hand. (Three sets of ten reps)

Quadricep Exercises
Exercise VI

Leg Press

Lie on a leg press machine, keeping your knees slightly bent, and release the bars located at the sides of the machine. Slowly lower the weight, bringing your knees into your chest. Then press the weight up by straightening your legs. Return to the start position to finish. (Three sets of ten reps)

Squats

Stand with your legs apart and your knees slightly bent. Lower your body until your thighs are parallel to the floor. When you reach a seated position reverse direction by straightening your legs until you are back at the start position. (Three sets of ten reps)

Lunge

Allow two dumbbells to hang down by your sides. Then take a long step with your right leg, and raise your left heel so that your left foot is on its toe. Slowly lower your body until your right foot is almost reaching the floor. Return to the start position. Repeat the same exercise with your left foot in front. (Three sets of ten reps on each foot)

Abdomenal Crunches
Exercise VII

Upper Frontal Abdomenal Workout

Lie on a padded surface with your knees bent and your fingers laced behind your head. Lift your head and shoulders off the ground with your chin separated about a fist's distance from your chest. Inhale while lifting up and exhale while returning to the floor. Perform ten crunches, followed by half a minute to rest. Begin with three sets of ten, gradually increasing to five sets of ten.

Lie on your back with your legs in the air, your knees slightly bent, and your hands beneath your head. Lift your upper body off the floor toward your knees as high as you can. Keep your head lifted just off your chest, and try to release the weight of your head onto your hands. Now perform ten small pulsing movements up and down. When finished, lower your head and legs to the floor and breath. Repeat this ten times with a few seconds rests between them. This is good for toning front abdominal muscle.

Lie on your back with your knees pulled in towards your chest and your arms behind your head. Lift your upper body off the floor and perform twenty small pulsing movements toward your knees and back. Now separate your knees into a wide position and do another twenty small pulses. Bring your knees together again and stretch them up straight towards the ceiling. Hold them steady and then perform twenty small pulses. Rest and then repeat all three exercises ten times. This exercises is good for toning your upper frontal abdominal muscles.

Lower Abdominal Muscles

Lie on the floor with your heels against the floor and your hands placed underneath your hips. Now raise one leg off the floor. Very slowly lower your leg while at the same time raising your other leg off the floor. Straighten your leg as much as possible. Keep your torso firmly pressed towards the floor. Swap the legs over twenty times and then rest. (Three sets)

Rope Crunch

Begin by kneeling in front of a high pulley machine with your body facing it. Grasp the rope attached to the pulley and keep your elbows in. Slowly curl your body downward, bringing your elbows toward your knees. Contract your abs, and then slowly return to the start position. (Three sets of ten reps)

Reverse Crunch

Begin by lying back on a flat surface. Curl your knees in toward your stomach and raise your butt as high as possible while keeping your upper back pressed to the surface. Contract your abs and then reverse directions, returning to the start position. (Three sets of ten reps)

Leg Lowering

Begin by lying on the floor with your hands at your sides and feet together. Extend your legs toward the ceiling and bring your lower body off the floor, starting with your lower back and proceeding to your mid-back. Then slowly roll back down in reverse sequence. (Three sets of ten pulses)

Twisting Crunch

Begin by lying face up on the floor with your calf resting on top of a flat bench. Your thighs should be perpendicular to the ground, and your hands should be folded across your chest. Slowly raise your shoulders up and forward toward your chest, then twist your body to the right. Feel the contraction in your abdominal muscles, and then slowly return to the start position. After twenty reps, repeat the same twist on your left side.

Flexibility Exercises

Over time muscles become stiffer and joints degenerate, producing less joint lubrication. Connective tissues gradually lose their elasticity and muscle fibers shorten. Approximately 80% of all lower back pain results from poorly coordinated muscles. By strengthening these joints and muscles, you could reduce your risk of injury. Remember, the stronger your core, the more you are able to execute more complicated exercises, loosen up your joints, and improve your overall flexibility.

Yoga Arch

Get down on all fours, resting on your hands and knees so that they are hip width apart. Lift your knees off the floor and straighten your legs. At the same time, arch your spine and lift your head upwards. Hold this for ten breaths, then release back on to your knees. Repeat this for ten reps. Make sure that you keep the abdominals working to lift your body so it does not sag. This exercise is good for spine flexibility and all the abdominal muscles.

Sit and Twist

Sit on the floor with your legs outstretched. Bend your left leg up toward your chest, cross it over your right leg and place your left foot flat on the floor. Turn your torso toward the knee and wrap your right arm around the upright leg. Pull your knee into your body so that you can feel the stretch. Hold the stretch for ten seconds, then release. Repeat the same process on the other side as well. Do this stretch for ten reps on each side.

Sit and Lean

Sit on the floor and bring your feet toward you so that the soles face each other and your legs are bent to either side of your body. Hold on to your ankles and slowly start to lean forward. As you lean forward, you will feel the top of your buttocks and the lower back start to stretch out. Lean as far forward as you can. Then bring yourself back to the upright position. Repeat twice, and try to lean slightly further the second time.

Lie and Lift

Lie on your back with your knees bent and your foot on the floor. Push your hips up into the air and hold the position for twenty seconds. Keep your hips as high as possible, and feel the stretch in your abdominals. Then return to the start position. (Ten reps)

Reach and Lie

Lie on your back, and extend your arms beyond your head. Press your heels into the floor, and stretch out as far as you can at both ends.

Back Strengtheners

Lie on your stomach with your palms on the floor. Slowly lift your chest off the floor by tightening your back muscles. Your arms and legs are used to provide stability. Repeat raising and lowering your chest to the floor, using only your back muscles. Do about ten lifts for five reps.

Lie and Lean

Lie on your back with your legs stretched. Bend your right knee, and hug the leg into your chest with your left arm. Stretch your right arm out on the floor to stabilize yourself. Now pull the right knee toward your left side, and hold it in the same position. Keep your knee pulled tight into your body. Hold for ten seconds, and then repeat the move on the other leg. Do this five times on each leg.

Stretch and Cool Down

After working out, you need to let those muscles stretch out and to give your body a rest. I suggest about five minutes or so to stretch and cool down after any physical exercise. Think of this cool down as a gift to your body and mind. Just as it's important to stretch before your work out, it is also important to stretch after your workout as well. Here are a few examples of stretches that you can use.

Deep Runner's Stretch

From a push-up position, place your right foot directly in between your hands, and place your knee in line with your foot. Stay in this pose for thirty seconds, and then repeat the same position on your other side.

Hamstring Stretch

Out of your runner's stretch (above), drive your hips high to the ceiling, keeping your hands on the floor. Next, straighten your legs gently and pull your toes up your front leg, toward your chin. You are going to feel a great stretch in the back of your leg. Stay in this position for thirty seconds, and then change legs.

Quad Stretch

Stand straight and bring the heel of your foot up toward your hamstrings, and hold it with the same arm. Hold this position for thirty seconds, and then change sides.

Seated Pike Stretch

Sit straight on a mat. Reach your arms high, and then lower your chest down to your quads. If you need to do it with a towel, you can place it on the bottom of your feet. Take a deep breath as you pull in your hamstrings and release your body, letting it go where it feels comfortable.

Upward Dog

Lie on your stomach; then lift your body with your elbows. Straighten your arms and lift your chest off the floor. Lift your chest so that your belly bottom comes off the floor, then lift the weight off your thighs as you look toward the ceiling.

Remember your stretching movement should be slow and controlled. Do not use force. As you hold the stretch and breathe, your muscles will relax and lengthen. Don't forget to breathe. Breathing is something that you don't think about because it's automatic, but it's an important component of any exercise routine. When you breathe correctly, you get enough oxygen in your system to increase your circulation and get the blood flowing to every part of your body, including your brain, making it easier to release the neurotransmitters that boost your mood and energy. Inhale through your nose and exhale slowly through your mouth.

De-Stress through Exercise

Stress evokes the fight or flight reaction by releasing into the body stress hormones designed to give us quick reactions, extra strength, and extra endurance. When we don't respond to the stress response by moving quickly or using our strength, our muscles stay tense, blood pressure stays high, breathing stays shallow, and all that cortisol and adrenaline courses through the body, causing all kinds of problems. Exercise changes the picture completely by allowing the body to expend energy.

Exercise also releases chemicals like beta endorphins that specifically counteract the effects of stress hormones, alerting the body that the danger has passed and now the relaxation response can begin. For example, exercises such as yoga and Pilates relax the body and the mind by helping connect movement to breath, which in turn stops the physical response of stress.

Yoga

There are many different types of yoga, but they all have common elements including the use of posture, breathing exercises, and meditation. Postures are practiced to strengthen and heal our body; breathing exercises help balance energy in the body; and meditation quiets the mind and centers us. For example, controlling our breathing enables us to control other functions of our body, such as heart rate, which causes blood pressure to distribute more oxygen to the body. It also keeps vital lung capacity from decreasing. There are many benefits to yoga. Primarily, it reduces stress and manages both depression and blood pressure. It strengthens every muscle in our body. It improves flexibility and promotes good posture, reducing back pain. And it enhances our concentration and mental focus.

Meditation

This is the practice of learning to be still. If you are driven by Reflexive Thinking (i.e. automatic thinking), learning to be still is just the ticket for proving that thoughts don't own you. From the beginning, your experience needs to be a positive one. Find a comfortable sitting position on the floor. Close your eyes or find a focus to look at. Try not to blink. Now bring your awareness to your breathing. Breathing acts as a hook for you to maintain a steady focus while trying to step apart from distracting thoughts. Breathe normally through your nose. You can incorporate a mantra to assist you in maintaining focus. A mantra is any word or phrase that your repeat with each breath. As you inhale, you form the mantra in your mind. Exhale and silently repeat your mantra. Keep slowly inhaling and exhaling. The only objective to focus on exclusively is your breath. You breathe in and out, nothing else. It sounds easy, but it's not. It takes a lot of practice to master it. If you get distracted, let the thoughts go and redirect your focus on your breathing. As you get more and more into it, you can start extending your time from ten minutes to thirty minutes or longer.

Pilates

This method of exercise works the whole body including the brain. Pilates is a series of exercises that focus on strengthening core postural muscles to support the spine for correct alignment. Pilates uses the resistance of the body to condition and correct itself with the goal of lengthening and aligning the spine. Both yoga and Pilates offer low-impact forms of strengthening and toning muscles while helping us get more in tune with our own bodies.

Final Suggestions

Stay hydrated. Water is important for your body. Without water, bodily processes necessary for life shut down in a matter of days. Water makes up 70% of your body's weight. Water has many functions. It acts as a lubricant all over the body. It provides sodium, calcium and magnesium to your body. It also contributes to temperature regulation, helps remove waste, and acts as a shock absorber in some parts of the body. You should drink eight to ten cups of water a day.

Rather than focusing on your negative energy (i.e. fatigue), you need to expand and enhance your awareness of your positive energy, of the level of energy experienced throughout the day. By concentrating on how tired you are, you only increase your fatigue. However, if you focus on how to create energy and act on it, your energy level will increase, promoting a higher level of vitality and physical and mental health. No matter how tired you feel, there is always a spark of energy in your body. You just need to get in touch with it and use it.

Any Physical Activity is Better than None

Exercising in bits and pieces throughout the day is just as effective as exercising all in one session. Throughout the day, you could walk up five or six flights of stairs instead of taking the elevator. You could play games like tag with your kids or grandkids. You could shovel your own snow or vacuum your house. Remember to turn off your T.V. and engage in any activity.

Now imagine that there is a new medication that relieves depression and anxiety with absolutely no harmful side effects. Imagine that this magical pill makes you feel more energized, stronger, healthier, puts you in a better mood, and makes your heart and brain work better. And imagine this pill is readily available to you. Would you want to try it? This pill is actually called "physical activity." Physical activity, unlike a pill, involves some effort, commitment, and a strong sense of exploration. But with all the added benefits, it's worth trying.

It's our natural state to be healthy and active. Premature aging is a disease that is greatly accelerated by a sedentary lifestyle and lack of physical activity. If you are living such a life, it is never too late to change. Take this chapter to heart and just make a decision to start moving more. It doesn't matter how old you are. It is never too late to improve your fitness. If you are in relatively good shape, then you will also benefit from increasing your activity level or just changing some of your routines. And if you are physically active and you like your routine, that's great: keep it up.

> "All parts of the body, if used in moderation and exercised in labors to which each is accustomed, become healthy, well developed, and age slowly; but if left unused and idle they become liable to disease, defective growth, and age quickly."
> Hippocrates

Hippocrates understood, some two-thousand five-hundred years ago, that an unused body resulted in loss of health and faster aging.

CHAPTER VI

Nutrition
Discover the Secrets of Healthy Eating

"To lengthen thy life, lessen thy meals."

Benjamin Franklin

Perhaps more than any other factor, nutrition plays an essential role in our overall health. The reason for this is simple: the food we eat effects virtually every cell, organ, and system in our bodies. We literally are what we eat. If we eat enough of the right foods, our bodies thrive and we stay healthy.

Healthy foods provide our cells with everything they need to function well, reproduce, and repair damage from a variety of sources. With the normal wear and tear of aging, our muscle mass decreases, our bones lose calcium and become weaker, and our metabolism slows down. Our collagen and our skin's elasticity decrease, and our heart rate declines, so it becomes even more important to equip ourselves with the necessary knowledge to enhance our health with proper nutrition to compensate for our losses.

We might think that just because we are in our fifties or sixties with all our years of experience, our food choices should be easier to make. But we are just as confused as ever. This confusion can turn us into unhealthy, emotional eaters, which could mean that we are eating not because we are hungry, but rather because we are stressed, depressed, bored, lonely, distracted, apathetic, or don't listen to the message our body sends to our brain signaling when we're hungry or full. The question we should ask ourselves is, would we fill up our gas tank when it's half empty? Probably not. So why would we eat when we are half full?

As we well know, none of us want to eat ourselves to a larger dress size, or make ourselves candidates for diabetes, heart problems, or early bone loss. But as we enter our middle-age years and our system undergoes many inevitable age-related changes, knowing which foods are health producing and which foods are damaging to our system becomes our major priority in life.

A lousy diet can be a springboard for a wide variety of age-related problems, including hypertension, diabetes, osteoporosis, and even cancer. But a simple change in our dietary habits can have remarkable effects on our health and on how we age. For most of us, simply eating less red meat and fatty foods and more fruits and vegetables can improve our health by reducing the amount of cholesterol in our system and giving our body the vitamins, minerals, and antioxidants it needs to function well and repair itself faster. This change in diet enables us to feel more energetic and have a greater sense of well-being.

This chapter is based on the same premise that flows throughout this book: a holistic approach to our well-being is essential. This means that our relationship with food is based not only on what we eat, when we eat, or how much we eat, but also on how we think about food and how we feel about ourselves and our self-image. Only after we understand these relationships can we move on to a healthier eating style. Our attitude toward food will change, and food will become our friend and partner on this important journey toward a healthier and more vigorous lifestyle. It will be lifestyle that is sustainable, practical, well balanced, and tasty.

Sustainable means that we can follow it for life. Balanced means that it has to include all three essential food groups: complex carbohydrates, proteins and fats. Practical means that we can create our own individualized plan that works best for us. And tasty means it has to include foods that we like, that we find satisfying and tasty.

What Type of Eater are You?

First, you need to understand your eating habits by recognizing your tendencies and triggers so you can sidestep them before they get you. There are a few reasons other than hunger that we eat such as boredom, stress, loneliness, depression, or just mindlessness.

Exercise I

Get in touch with the reasons you eat by answering the following questions.

1. Do you eat when you are under stress? When faced with many problems at once do you find yourself eating more?
2. Do you eat mindlessly throughout the day? Are you always nibbling on something throughout the day and night?
3. Are you a social eater? Do you eat more when out with friends?
4. Are you an "on the run" eater? Do you constantly grab something and run?
5. Are you an emotional eater? Do you eat when feeling some kind of void?
6. Does food preoccupy your thoughts?
7. Do you pre-plan for your daily meals?
8. Do you follow any type of diet?
9. Do you eat the same type of foods?

If your answers are mostly "yes," then you react to strong emotions such as stress, sadness, frustration, or even joy. You reach for food for what might be the wrong reasons, not because you're hungry, but rather to fulfill your emotional needs. Think before you eat and consider whether you are hungry or trying to fill a void that is not in your tummy. This is a good time to become aware of your relationship with food.

Examining the reasons why we eat when we do is the first step in the process of becoming cognizant of our eating patterns. Many of us might expect that our hunger drives would match our need for energy, so we would naturally consume fewer calories if we needed fewer calories. But this is not necessarily so. For example, we might eat because we are tired, stressed, depressed, lonely, bored, or mindless. Many times we eat when we are not hungry, or we eat more than we need. We choose big portion sizes and we finish them without paying attention to whether we are full or not. Being aware of why we eat when we're not hungry or why we always feel hungry at a specific time of day helps us better understand our relationship with food and allows us to make the necessary changes in our eating behavior.

The act of mindfully enjoying healthy and sustaining food is one of the simplest and most powerful ways to nourish ourselves on a daily basis. We honor hunger, respect fullness, and enjoy the pleasure of eating. Optimal nourishment involves eating the right amount and type of food as well as understanding that our metabolic processes are influenced by our emotional state, genetic make up, macronutrient intake (vitamins and minerals), exercise, and environment. Nourishing ourselves means paying attention to each of these areas.

Our emotional state is influenced by many factors, including our body-image, anxiety level, stress, fatigue, depression, anger, fear, and perceptions. For example, self-respect and self-acceptance are at the roots of our body image. Regardless of how we feel right now, the first step toward optimal health is to have respect for our bodies.

Respecting one's body was found by psychologists and physicians to create a metabolic milieu that is conducive to our optimal fat burning, while unresolved emotional stress keeps excess body fat firmly in place because the stress hormones cortisol and adrenaline drastically affect our metabolism.

Most of us have experienced our weight going up or down when we are upset. Our need to eat more when we are emotionally upset can cause us to gain weight. But this weight gain might serve as a defense mechanism against the pain that our stress is causing. The first step in changing this route is by honestly examining how and why we use food to soothe ourselves.

For example, many of us crave sugar when we're upset. These sugar cravings become our survival mechanism to fight changes in our mood and anxiety level. We call this type of eating "emotional eating." The underlying causes of emotional eating are called "the antecedent," something that precedes our eating when we're not hungry. The antecedent can be a stressful event, a negative thought, feelings of anger, irritation, loneliness, or boredom.

The antecedent is always followed by consequences such as eating to make ourselves feel better. Food becomes a tranquilizer that calms our nerves and fills our emotional void. Using food to solve our emotional problems is not a long term solution. It's a temporary one that masks the real reasons we eat in the first place. One major lesson that we all need to learn is to eat when we are truly hungry by listening to the messages our body sends to our brain. In other words, we need to pay close attention to our mind-body connection.

Our emotional state is also influenced by "our diet mentality." Dieters avoid food the whole day, eat only dinner, and are so hungry that they gulp whatever is available. Once we get into this unhealthy routine, we stop our bodies from functioning properly. When we decide to skip breakfast, we are actually sabotaging ourselves because our metabolism is not working until we have our first meal.

Breakfast is the most important meal of the day because it sets the stage for our blood sugar for the rest of the day. Research has shown that eating a low fat and high fiber breakfast can result in a lower fat intake for the entire day, which helps our metabolism use the fat already stored in our bodies for energy. It also improves our memory, reduces the risk of high cholesterol, decreases insulin resistance, and keeps our blood sugar levels stable, reducing hunger cravings. Eating lean protein, healthy carbs, fruits and vegetables, and whole grains is a perfect way to start the day.

Your Relationship with Food

It's important to recognize that our relationship with food was developed early in our lives. Strong messages were passed down from our families and significant adults. From our mothers, we have internalized messages about personal weight and food history. What kind of relationship did our mothers have with food? What was your mother's own eating philosophy? Did she pay attention to what she ate? How much did she eat? How frequently did she eat? Did she pay attention to what you ate? How much you ate? How frequently you ate? Once we become aware of these strong messages that we have internalized throughout our childhood years and beyond, we will be able to better understand our present eating habits.

In my case, food was a symbol that represented my mother's love and nurturance. Being a Holocaust survivor, my mother instilled in me the high value of food. For her, wasting food was unacceptable since she experienced extreme deprivation in the concentration camp. I have internalized these strong message from her which said, "I made this food for you because I love you." Even today with my grandchildren, this pattern repeats itself. Cooking their favorite meals means I love them, and their eating them means they love me.

We might have learned early in life that food can ease our anger, fear, and upset feelings. However, this pattern of behavior continues throughout our lives since we have never learned to trust these painful feelings and realize that eventually they will pass.

Addictive eating is not a condition to be controlled by willpower. Rather, it's a condition that we adopt early in our lives. Some of the signs to watch for are eating when not hungry, a constant preoccupation with food, feeling guilty after overeating, enjoying eating alone, repeatedly failing at dieting, and eating to escape stress and loneliness.

To change these behaviors, we need to be aware of why we eat in the first place and ask ourselves if we are hungry, depressed, tired, lonely, or stressed. We need to identify the causes for bad eating habits and be aware of how stress-related eating is at the core of our bad behavior.

Let's remember that behind all our self-sabotaging behavior is the critical voice that encourages us to eat unhealthy. We need to challenge that voice and change it to a healthy voice that encourages us to stay on our plan and achieve our goals. We need to stop our self-sabotaging talk that tells us, "I can't do this," "I always fail," "It's too hard," "I'm too old," "I'm not quite ready," "Maybe in a few weeks…" We need to become a true partner on our quest toward a healthy life.

Exercise II

The following exercises will help you get in touch with your eating personality, your relationship with food, and your body image.

The first part of this exercise will help you get in touch with the relationship that exists between your eating habits and your moods. By answering the next few questions, you will be able to discover this important connection. The second part of this exercise will help you practice these connections.

1. What feelings or moods do you associate with eating?
2. Do you eat more when you are stressed, tired, angry, or lonely?

3. Do you eat the same amount or less when you are calm?
4. Do you eat more at specific times of the day?
5. Do you feel fatigue at certain points of the day?
6. Do you eat more or the same amount when you eat alone?
7. Do you eat more or less when you eat with others?
8. What types of foods do you associate with your mood swings?
9. Does your eating pattern fluctuate?
10. Do you eat while watching T.V., talking on the phone, reading, or doing different chores?

Practice

Try this at your next meal. Sit down to eat and look at your food. Bring your full attention to where you are, how you feel, and what thoughts are going through your head. Notice everything about your food: its presentation, smell, color, texture, shape, and so on. Utilize all of your senses to get in touch with the food that you're about to eat. As you take the first bite, begin to chew slowly. Simply eat. Be attentive only to the activity of eating, and notice how satisfied or dissatisfied you are with your food. Don't watch T.V., read, or speak on the phone. Notice what you experience as you eat. Pay attention to your feelings, your thoughts, your mood, and so on. Practicing mindful eating will help you get in touch with your senses, feelings, thoughts, and emotions associated with your meal. It will help you realize why you eat in the first place. Are you hungry, bored, tired, or just thoughtlessly eating?

Your Body Image

Exercise III

This exercise will help you gain awareness of your body-image.

Look in a full-length mirror and ask yourself: "Do I like the way I look? What do I like about my body? What would I like to change? Do

I want to eat healthier? Do I want to feel more energized? Do I want to increase my stamina?" Be open and honest with your answers.

Accept who you are today in the mirror, and only then can you start changing. By accepting who you are right now, you give yourself permission to change. Be honest and don't pretend that you are more in control of your body than you really are. If you do that, you are creating an obstacle to achieving your goal. Only after you accept your body are you ready to give yourself permission to change what you don't like about yourself. Remember, any obstacles undermine your ability to change your eating habits. Once you accept both your positive and negative body images you are ready to move on.

Your Current Eating Philosophy

Exercise IV

Start by keeping a diary of your current eating and drinking habits. Put down everything you put in your mouth. Keep on doing this exercise for a few weeks or until you feel in control of your eating habits. Record all of the following:

How much do you eat and drink each day? (Include all meals and snacks.)

What do you eat and drink each day? (Include all types of foods and drinks.)

How hungry are you every time you eat?

What times of the day do you get hungry?

What time of the day do you feel tired or low in energy?

How do you feel every time you put something in your mouth?

What is your physical state every time you eat?

Do you eat more when you are tired or stressed?

What do you eat when tired?

What do you eat when relaxed?

Quiz on Major Food Groups

Exercise V

This exercise will help you find out what you currently know about the three major food groups. Learning about all the food groups as well as the proper combination of foods will serve you as an important guide towards your quest for healthy eating.

Each of the foods listed below belongs to one food category: carbohydrates, proteins, or fats. For each of the following words, write down the food group that it belongs too: margarine, banana, potato, steak, yogurt, corn, chick peas, green beans, canola oil, bread, egg, farmer cheese, avocado, tofu, spaghetti, bread, rice, orange juice, milk, olive oil. *Don't look at the answers below.*

Fat: margarine, canola oil, avocado, olive oil.

Carbohydrate: banana, spaghetti, bread, rice, yogurt, orange juice, corn, chick peas, green beans, milk, potato.

Protein: steak, egg, farmer cheese, tofu.

This short quiz is a good test of your knowledge about the three major food groups. Look at your answers closely, and see how much you know so far about different foods. If you know them all, good for you. If you are confused about some foods, start learning about them as you read through this chapter.

Plan for Change

Would you like to improve what you eat, how much you eat, how frequently you eat, or decrease the unhealthy foods that you eat? There are many other goals that you can set for yourself. Choose one that you can accomplish. Don't set yourself up for failure.

Make a plan for yourself for every day of the week. Start with simple goals. Do not take upon yourself more than you can do for that week. Once you see yourself as being successful, you will gain more courage to continue with bigger goals. There is a significant power in making a written plan and sticking with it.

If you encounter obstacles, you need to reexamine your plan and make changes as needed. Sometimes reviewing your goals and changing them might work better for you at this moment in your life.

Know Your Food Groups

More than any other factor, nutrition can accelerate our aging process, or it can slow it down. In our middle adulthood, eating healthy foods serves as a counterbalance for the normal wear and tear that comes with age. We need good nutrients to keep healthy and strong.

In our young adulthood, our body's own maintenance and repair system kept compensating for the effects of both normal and excessive wear and tear. But as we age, our body's repair system slows down, and we can feel the effects of our system's wear and tear more profoundly. For example, when we are younger our hormones work together to regulate many of our body's functioning. As we age though, the levels of our hormones decrease. Our hormonal clock gets out of sync, resulting in a decline of our body's functioning. Our growth hormones that help us form muscle mass decline considerably. Our estrogen, testosterone, and thyroid hormones, which are all important for regulating our body's functioning, will drop drastically.

Another age-related problem that we encounter is the accumulation of free-radicals in our bodies that attack our collagen and elastin, two proteins that keep our skin flexible and moist. Furthermore, the slowing down of our metabolism, which is our life force, and the decrease in our muscle mass and loss of bone density could cause osteoporosis.

The question is "How do we keep our body functioning well into middle age, and what type of nutrition does it need?

Healthy Nutrition

One of the most effective ways to keep our bodies functioning well is by consuming a lot of foods high in water content. The two major foods groups in this category are fruits and vegetables. Fruits and vegetables contain 70% water, meaning they are easy to digest, and our body does not have to work hard, which results in much less energy consumed.

Fruits have the highest water content, approximately 80 to 90%, which is important for cleaning our bodies. They also have a high concentration of vitamins, minerals, fatty acids, and good carbohydrates—all essentials for our body's needs. Fruits can be looked at as our body's cleansing food because they pass through our body very fast.

Eating different color fruits is beneficial for our health. They boost the antioxidant levels in our bodies and keep our brain young, our bones strong, our heart functioning well, and our metabolism fired up. Several studies have found that eating food rich in antioxidants like fruits and vegetables significantly reduces the risk of developing cognitive impairment.

Vegetables are another important food group that we can consume as much as we need. Because vegetables have less carbs and lots of fiber, it takes the body a longer time to digest them. They fill us up, but they have very few calories and no fat. Studies show that leafy greens have a lot of powerful nutrients and vitamins that are essential for our body's proper functioning. For example, spinach and kale are both packed with iron and vitamins A, B, and E. Lettuce is high in magnesium, potassium, and vitamins A and E.

Since vegetables are known to be high in fiber, they offer a few important benefits. Firstly, they fill us up, so we don't get hungry that fast. They hold water in our stomach. They are digested slowly. Some of their calories are eliminated unabsorbed, and they have a low caloric density. We can eat a lot of them for a small amount of calories. They are generally bulky and contain a lot of water. Vegetables also include chemicals that are essential to our immune system, muscle and brain functioning, and our bone and heart health. For example, dark leafy greens are high in calcium, magnesium, potassium, zinc, fiber, folic acid, and vitamins A, C and E.

Vitamins E and C and beta-carotene are important antioxidants that fight free-radicals accumulating in our bodies. Even though free-radical damage begins at birth, in a younger body the damage is relatively minor and easier to repair. With age, however, the accumulated effects of free-radical damage begin to take their toll. For example, free radicals attack our collagen and elastin that keep our skin flexible and moist. By feeding ourselves antioxidants, we can give ourselves a powerful health burst.

Vitamin E could be found in fatty foods such as, nuts, seeds, whole grains, and wheat germs. This vitamin is important for our brain's functioning, our arteries, and our immune system.

Vitamin C offers protection of our arteries by increasing our good cholesterol (HDL) and reducing our bad cholesterol (LDL). It boosts our immune system functioning by hiking our body's level of antioxidants. Vitamin C can be found in fruits and vegetables such as oranges, cantaloupes, sweet peppers, strawberries, broccoli, tomatoes, and all citrus fruits.

Beta-carotene is another powerful antioxidant that protects our cells by snuffing out free-radicals. It prevents heart attacks by keeping our arteries from clogging, and it stimulates our immune functioning. Beta-carotene can be found in fruits and vegetables, such as carrots, sweet potatoes, spinach, kale, winter squash, tomatoes, and bell peppers.

Eating a lot of antioxidant rich foods like vegetable, fruits, olive oil, seeds, nuts, almonds, whole grains, and beans is a good way to keep our bodies healthy. We can also benefit by taking a supplement of vitamin C, D, and beta-carotene once a day.

As we age, we all complain that our metabolism slows down. Our metabolism is our life force. The key to our health is maintaining a good balance of our interrelated metabolic processes: oxidation and inflammation. Oxidation is important because it combines our food with oxygen to create energy. But excess oxidation causes free radical damage. The most common causes of free radical damage are smoking, poor eating habits, environmental toxins, inflammation, and excess sun exposure. Eating a lot of antioxidant-rich foods is a good counterbalance for all these toxicities.

Inflammation is another metabolic process that we need to keep under control. Inflammation is the essential tool of our immune system to fight off germs, but high amounts of inflammation can be the cause of many chronic diseases and premature aging. An important agent to fight inflammation is methylation, which protects our body from all types of poison. This is the process our body uses to neutralize toxicity. The best support for this metabolic process are the vitamin B, B6 and B12, and folic acid. We can find all these vitamins in foods such as beans, lean meats, fruits, vegetables, nuts, legumes, fish, and non-fat dairy .

We can also increase our metabolic rates by eating regularly and exercising. To maintain our metabolic level we need to eat regular meals: breakfast, lunch, dinner and two snacks. By restricting our calories we actually slow down our metabolic rate. By eating three meals and two snacks a day we help regulate our digestive system and keep our blood sugar steady. Having a healthy breakfast that includes proteins, high quality carbs, and unsaturated fats fires up our metabolism and keeps us functioning well throughout the day. Having proteins with each meal increases our metabolism by helping maintain and build muscle mass.

Eating healthy foods, such as lean proteins, chicken, turkey, fish, egg whites, fat-free yogurt, beans, lentils, peas, tofu, soybeans; high quality carbs like brown rice, whole grains, barley and quinoa; as well as healthy fats rich in Omega-3 fatty acids form the basis for our overall health and well-being.

Another major task that we face in middle-adulthood is keeping our bone density and muscle mass from rapidly decreasing. We can accomplish this by increasing our intake of calcium, vitamin D, and magnesium. Between the ages of 40 and 60, our bone density begins to decrease. The major causes are menopause, weight loss, and eating disorders. Our estrogen level plummets, which means we may be at risk of osteoporosis as estrogen regulates bone loss.

Lack of exercise and insufficient calcium and vitamin D in our diet accelerates our bone loss and muscle-mass deterioration. As a result of losing muscle mass, our fat increases. The best way to fight this is through healthy eating and regular exercise. Those of us who are prone to osteoporosis commonly lack the necessary nutrients found in fruits, vegetables, beans, nuts, seeds, salmon, legumes, whole grains, fat-free dairy products, and other foods that are high in calcium and anti-inflammatory proteins.

Vitamin D boosts our body's ability to absorb calcium. We can get vitamin D from foods such as, fruits, vegetables, nuts, seeds, eggs, spinach, kale, salmon, tuna, cod, halibut, sea bass, salmon, whole grains, and all dark green leafy vegetables.

The best sources that provide us with **calcium** are yogurt, milk, soymilk, tofu, broccoli, kale, soybeans, and almonds. Remember, calcium is useless without vitamin D. Vitamin D allows calcium to move from our gastrointestinal tracks to the parts of our body that need it—mainly our bones.

Including **healthy proteins** with our meals is also important for the health of our bones. Research studies have shown that those of us who don't eat enough proteins have reduced calcium absorption, lower bone density, and higher rates of bone loss. The best sources for healthy proteins are fish, skinless chicken and turkey, eggs, beans, lentils, fat free dairy, yogurt, tofu, nuts, seeds, and big quantities of green leafy vegetables.

Simple carbohydrates, another age promoter in our bloodstream, attacks our arteries, drains our energy, raises our blood pressure, and in some cases causes diabetes. Simple carbs provide instant energy because their small molecules are digested quickly, giving us an immediate bust of energy as well as a rise in our blood sugar. Most processed foods and foods prepared with refined sugar are simple carbs. These include white flour pasta, white rice, breads, cakes and juices, just to name a few. These types of carbohydrates are digested quickly, raise our blood sugar to an unhealthy level, and are turned to glucose by our body.

Glucose is our primary source of energy. Keeping our blood sugar level fairly balanced is one of the highest priorities of our metabolism. When our blood sugar gets too low we become tired and dizzy. When our blood sugar level gets too high, it makes our blood sticky, which is bad for our cells. Our cells became starved for oxygen and nutrients, which can cause big damage, including diabetes.

Most **complex carbohydrates**, including fruits, vegetables, beans, and whole grains have low glycemic loads triggering only a small rise in our blood sugar. On the other hand, refined pulverized grain has a high glycemic load which causes a high rise in our blood sugar. The steeper the drop, the worse we will feel. That's why low-quality carbs can lead to feeling irritable, depressed, and sluggish.

If we eat low-quality carbs regularly our blood sugar won't have a chance to stabilize and neither will our mood. That's why limiting sugary and refined foods in our diet is important for both our physical and mental health. To stay on an even keel all day, our meals and snacks should combine high quality carbs with good proteins. Protein is critical because it's an important stabilizer. It does not add to blood sugar, but instead it helps slow the absorption of carbohydrates from our blood.

Most of us are amazed by how much better we feel when we eliminate most refined foods, excess sugar, and starch from our daily consumption. For example, when we eat high-glycemic index carbohydrates, which in general are starchy and sugary foods, our bodies quickly metabolize them into sugar, which causes a spike in our insulin level. But when we eat low-glycemic index carbohydrates, our bodies break them down slowly, which means our blood sugar and our insulin levels stay relatively steady over a long period of time.

The most important key to lifelong weight maintenance and good health is knowing how to keep our blood sugar stable. Foods such as candy, soda, white bread, rice, white potatoes, white pasta, and cake, raise our blood sugar quickly and signal to our pancreas to release the hormone insulin. Insulin is a storage hormone that takes our sugar out of the blood and stores it in our cells until it can be burned as fuel. If this energy is not used right away, then it gets stored as fat. Stable blood sugar results from eating the right amount of protein, the right kind of carbohydrates, and the right amounts of fat.

Fiber is another important food group. High fiber foods are one of our best longevity weapons. Years of research have found that the more fiber we eat, the better our health and weight become. Fiber helps us feel full longer, so we don't get to munch one hour after dinner. Fiber also slows the absorption of food into our bloodstream, which helps balance our blood sugar and lowers our risk for diabetes as well as keeps our digestive tract moving and reducing our cholesterol level.

High Fiber Foods

Fruits: avocado, blueberries, strawberries, apples

Vegetables: carrots, corn, artichoke, baked potatoes with skin

Whole grain foods: multigrain beads, muffins, pasta, brown rice, whole grain ready to eat cereals without added sugar, barley, polenta, quinoa, whole grain couscous

Whole Grains and Legumes

Some good legumes are beans, chickpeas, fava beans, black beans, lentils, red kidney beans, and lima beans as well as nuts and seeds including walnuts, almonds, hazelnuts, pine nuts, peanuts, pistachios, cashew, pecans, and all type of seeds. Grains, legumes, nuts and seeds are delicious, filling, and rich sources of proteins, fiber, and vitamins. They provide us with iron, dietary fiber, and vitamins E and B-complex. Because our bodies absorb these foods slowly, they provide sustained energy and help keep our blood sugar levels steady.

Dietary Fats make up a major food group that is important for our body's healthy functioning. Fats transport oxygen to our cells. They are an important component for building cells and body tissue as well as absorbing vitamins and other nutrients to keep us healthy. There are two kinds of fats: unsaturated (healthy) fats and saturated (unhealthy) fats. Healthy fats are important to a good eating plan because the solid weight of our brain is 60% fat!

But we need to be aware of the delicate balance of these fats in our food. Foods that are high in Omega-3 fatty acids are the best. Omega-3's found in fatty fish, such as salmon, tuna, mackerel, and sardines keep our arteries young. They lower our bad cholesterol levels, raise our good cholesterol, improve our heart functioning by regulating our heart beats, make aging arteries more flexible, help block inflammatory processes that promote arthritis and diabetes, and restore our artery elasticity. The more fish oil in our body's cells, the less clogged and aged our arteries are. Foods such as salmon, tuna, avocados, walnuts, and green leafy vegetables are the best source of Omega-3 fatty acid. Omega-3 fatty acid is our miracle nutrient. It supports our immune system, reduces our bad cholesterol level, strengthens our bones, and improves our brain functioning since our brain itself is built from Omega-3 fatty acids.

Unsaturated fats are found in most vegetable oils, especially olive oil, nuts, leafy green vegetables, fatty fish such as salmon, mackerel, sardines, and tuna as well as nuts like almonds, cashews, pecans, seeds, and walnuts.

The other type of fats are the saturated fats. They are important to our body's proper functioning because they protect our liver from common toxins and lower lipoprotein, which is a key substance in our blood that indicates proneness to heart disease. Our bodies need saturated fats in order to properly utilize the other fats in our diet, especially the important Omega-3's. Omega-3 fats are better retained in our tissues when we incorporate saturated fats in our meal. The most common saturated fats are found in butter, milk, coconut oil, goat milk, cow milk, all fatty red meats, vegetable shortening, and fast foods, especially fried foods.

Diets that are high in saturated fats, trans fats, and omega-6 fats have been linked to insulin resistance, accumulation of triglyceride (bad cholesterol), and plaque in our arteries. Therefore, there is an important need for a healthier ratio between our Omega-3's and Omega-6's in our daily nutritional plan. The ratio should be 2:1. To improve our ratio we need to switch from vegetable oils to olive oil, flax oil, or canola oil; consume more fish; consume more nuts, walnuts and dark leafy vegetables; limit fatty red meats and replace them with skinless chicken, turkey, veal and lamb.

Spices and herbs maximize nutrient density, they naturally increase our metabolism, and they also add flavor to our food. Most of the time they help us curtail the use of salt, resulting in less bloating and water retention. Without too much salt, our overall health improves, especially if we suffer from high blood pressure. If we use more spices in our food, we will lose the cravings for salty snacks, and our taste palate will change. To give our food good taste, we can use different herbs and spices, such as rosemary, thyme, sage, oregano, fennel, garlic, cloves, bay leaves, mustard, cilantro, and cinnamon. As a result, we will develop our own individual taste buds. Herbs and spices are known to boost our metabolism for efficient calorie burning. Studies have found that some of these seasonings triple our body's ability to burn calories for fuel, rather than store them as fat.

There is also a need to develop a sensible salt consumption since high salt intake has been linked to high blood pressure, tension, heart attacks, and even stroke. Yet salt is so widely used in cooking that, unless we cook our own food from fresh and natural sources, we are likely to be exposed to salt without knowing it. Salt consumption is a hard habit to break. Salt actually dulls our sense of taste, which means that over time, we will be reaching for that salt shaker more often to get the flavor we desire from our food. Some good alternatives to salt are sea salt, kelp, and miso.

Staying away from artificial sweeteners is important because they are made of a mix unnatural chemicals that our bodies cannot process well. A healthier choice is stevia, which comes from a sweet leaf, honey, and pure maple syrup. Natural sweeteners strengthen our immune system and aid antioxidant functions.

Tea is one of the greatest secrets of stopping aging. Tea has been known as an extraordinary anti-aging drink for thousands of years in Asian culture. Until recently most research hailed green tea as the strongest in antioxidants and best to protect us from heart disease. However, new research has uncovered the important benefits that our bodies get from all types of teas, including white tea, oolong tea, and black tea. Caffeine found in tea and coffee, when consumed in moderation, can lower depression and stimulate our central nervous system by increasing the activity of our brain chemical dopamine, our reward and pleasure center. Drinking tea is also beneficial for our health because it flushes from our system the toxic foods that we eat, speeds up our metabolism, and improves our overall health.

Make Hydration a Priority

Water is essential to our cellular functioning. It regulates body temperature, lubricates joints, assists in elimination of waste, and protects our body tissues. Approximately 60% of our weight is water. Every system in our body depends on water to function. We need to consume eight to ten cups of water daily.

When we are dehydrated, our body temperature increases, and we lose not only water but also electrolytes, essential minerals, potassium, and sodium, which are important for our body's healthy functioning. Dehydration warning signs include dizziness, headaches, weakness, and dry mouth. We cannot replace the health benefits of drinking water by substituting beverages such as soft drinks, coffee, or juices.

If our bodies are not sufficiently hydrated, our metabolism will become depressed. When our metabolism slows down, food has a tendency to turn into fat, and we become much more fatigued. Water is also vital for cleaning our colon, absorbing and transporting nutrients, and flushing out waste products, including fat and toxins.

Healthy food fuels cell growth and regeneration. What we eat on a daily basis directly affects the health of our brains and bodies. Proper nutrition is the key to our staying healthy. For example, we can notice the effects of our mood and energy level after a meal. Food can make us feel great, energized, sleepy, tired, inactive, or distractible. So let's watch our calorie intake, increase good fats and decrease bad fats, increase good carbs and decrease bad carbs, eliminate artificial sweeteners, reduce salt intake, plan healthy snacks and have regular meals.

Customize Your Eating Plan

It's important that you eat every four hours, which means you will probably be eating five times a day. You should basically eat three meals and two snacks. If you don't eat frequently, you get too hungry, which might trigger your old behaviors and bad food decisions. When you eat frequently and healthily, you actually increase your metabolism, making your body burn more calories, while at the same time you feel more balanced. Often those dips in energy or mood that you feel at certain points of the day are caused by drops in your blood sugar. Avoid those drops by eating regularly. Create your own individualized eating plan that allows you to take control over your life and be in charge of your own food consumption. There is a feeling of empowerment when you create your own eating plan and stick to it.

Steps to Follow

Exercise VI

1. Listen to your appetite. Your body sends the message to your brain: "I am hungry." Listen and honor that message by eating when you are hungry and stopping when you feel satisfied. By not filling yourself up, you allow your digestive power to work at an optimal level.
2. Pay attention and stop the distractions around you when you eat. Turn off the T.V., don't take any phone calls, and avoid other activities like reading or working. Protect your meal time so you can enjoy your food in a relaxed manner.
3. Use food to feed your body, not your emotions. It's easy to resort to food when you feel tired, stressed, bored, or anxious. Unfortunately, if you are trying to fill an emotional void in your life, you will not be very successful and the calories will be stored as fat. Use food to satisfy the energy your body needs to function well.
4. Start with a simple goal that you can accomplish. For example, improve what, how much, or how frequently you eat. Or try decreasing some of the unhealthy foods that you eat. There are many goals that you can set for yourself, but don't set yourself up for failure.
5. Make a plan for yourself for every day of the week. Do not take upon yourself more than you can do for that week. Once you see yourself as having been successful it will give you more courage to continue with bigger goals. You

will gain confidence that will help you achieve the rest of your goals. You will see big changes in your energy level, mood, and overall physical and mental wellbeing.

6. Practice, practice, practice until you feel comfortable with your achievement and then move on to your next goal. If you encounter obstacles, re-examine your plan, and make the necessary changes as needed.

7. Create your own energy throughout the day with your food choices by finding a balance between clean protein, complex carbs, and good fats at every meal. Fight fatigue and increase your metabolism.

8. Keep a daily plan. Once you've done it for a few weeks, you might not need to write everything down. It will become a habit. Throughout the first few weeks, adjust your plan as needed. Be kind to yourself, and take into account that sometimes you might deviate from your meal plan. Do not punish yourself; just go back to it. It's okay to give yourself permission to have a cheat meal from time to time. It does not mean that you are regressing. Have confidence in your abilities to follow through. I know that you will feel more energetic and younger within a short period of time.

9. Make health, not weight loss, your goal. Enjoy your newfound experience of eating healthy, and associate the experience of reaching a healthy weight with healthy eating choices.

Summary of Foods that Revitalize Your Body and Mind

Exercise VII

1. Favor foods rich in complex carbohydrates, such as whole grain products.

2. Eat four to five servings of fresh fruits each day.

3. Eat five to six servings of fresh or frozen vegetables. Choose a variety of green and yellow vegetables.

4. Choose vegetable sources of protein, including beans, legumes, seeds, nuts, and tofu.
5. Use nonfat or low-fat dairy products.
6. Minimize your intake of red meats by replacing them with fish, chicken, turkey, veal, and lamb.
7. Keep hydrated with eight to ten glasses of water.
8. Limit the coffee intake to no more then two cups a day. Try to substitute tea for coffee.
9. Use olive oil for cooking.
10. Increase your fiber rich foods, which can help you in normalizing elimination and lowering your cholesterol levels.
11. Make your health a top priority.
12. Enjoy your food. Savor the texture, flavor, and color of your food choices. Watch portion sizes, and balance your food intake with your activity level. Drink lots of water. Exercise, rest, and relax. These three important lifestyle components can greatly affect your eating habits.

This chapter helped you familiarize yourself with good nutrition and its important health benefits. But it's up to you to follow through and apply them for the rest of your life. A helpful tool on this journey toward a healthy eating style is listening to your body, which simply means paying attention to your cravings, to the way things taste, to the feeling inside your mouth, and to your sense of hunger or satiety. Sometimes you might be eating long after your hunger is satisfied, just out of habit, nervousness, loneliness, or anger. By honoring your appetites and cravings, you will actually make healthy eating easier.

I hope that the information provided in this chapter will inspire you to make healthy food choices. Your body its remarkable, so feed it with high quality foods that it deserves and needs. If your body does not feel the full range of nutrition it needs for energy and maintenance, over time it will fail to run efficiently, and it will age prematurely.

"The rest of the world lives to eat, I eat to live."

Socrates

Part II

CHAPTER VII

A Holistic Approach to Your Outer Anim-Morphosis (Skin, Hair, and Teeth)

> "Think of what you have rather than what you lack. Of the things you have, select the best and then reflect how eagerly you would have sought them, if you did not have them."
>
> Marcus Aurelius

The first part of this book focused on improving your *self*, by strengthening your self-awareness and self-acceptance, improving your physical and mental stamina with daily activities, improving your eating habits and your overall wellbeing by learning about health-promoting foods, and learning about the damaging effects that stress has on your body and mind. You have learned that by enhancing and strengthening your inner self, you can change your thoughts (i.e. eliminate irrational thought), your beliefs, habits and behaviors, as well as your critical voice that puts you down and hinders your growth. You have learned the importance of unconditional self-acceptance as well as the need to celebrate all that you have instead of dwelling on everything you don't have.

You have learned about the strong interconnection that exists between your inner and outer life. This interconnection sets the foundation for both your mental and physical wellbeing. One cannot survive without the other, and everything that your inner self needs your outer self needs as well. Simply put, the way you feel is the way you look, and the way you look is the way you feel. Your feelings are clearly reflected on your face, body, and your general health. If you feel depressed, your face will look pale and saggy, and your body will be void of energy. But if you feel good, your face will look bright, and your body will be energized.

A number of questions remain. How can you create and keep a healthy balance between your inner and outer self? What happens if this equilibrium is disrupted? What happens when you place more emphasis on your outer self while neglecting your feelings? These are some of the questions that the second part of this book addresses. This is your time to create an overall healthy lifestyle at this crucial point of your life: middle age.

The first part of this book focused on how to improve our inner health with healthy eating, exercising, keeping our brain active, de-stressing, and having eight hours of sleep. The same argument is reintroduced when dealing with our ability to maintain our outer appearance, including our skin, hair, teeth, and nails. We need to follow the same healthy lifestyle to maintain a youthful and healthy look. But most importantly, our outer health is a clear expression of our unique personality, which guides the way we treat our body and establish our state of mind. Just as your eyes are the window to your soul, your skin is the window to your body's health.

If we eat healthily and are active both physically and mentally, our skin and hair glow, we feel fit, we have more energy, and we feel better about ourselves. If we eat unhealthily and are inactive our skin and hair becomes dull and lifeless, our energy level drops, and we feel tired, depressed, and unhappy. So our general self-care effects our state of mind as well as our self-image. This strong interconnection that exists between our inner and outer self is at the core of our existence, which means that our skin, hair, nails, and teeth have a dynamic interaction with the health of the rest of our body, and they must be toned in the same way that we tone our muscles. A frail body is equated with frail skin, and a healthy body is equated with a glowing skin.

Your Skin

Our skin, like the rest of our body, undergoes many changes throughout our lifetime. But these changes vary greatly from person to person depending on heredity, eating habits, sun exposure, smoking and drinking habits, stress, and other lifestyle choices. In our twenties and thirties, our skin is soft and strong thanks to the combination of collagen, elastin, lubricating oils, and moisture. As we age, our dermis, the middle layer of our skin, becomes thinner, resulting in a loss of collagen. The loss of collagen, which is the most important protein that keeps our skin healthy looking, results in sagging and, over time, wrinkling. Usually women show signs of aging before men because our skin gets thinner and dryer earlier in our lives.

During the past fifty years, the cosmetics industry has convinced us to rely on the magical power of its products to stop the natural progression of aging. As a result, we have relinquished our responsibility to take care of our body, mind, and beauty. We relinquished our powers over our own body's ability to preserve and improve our looks as well as our health and followed the guidelines set by our culture. Our culture teaches us to rely on the magical powers of creams, capsules, and procedures rather than our body's own ability to preserve our healthy looks.

Inside our body, we have enormous powers to rejuvenate our skin, hair, teeth, and nails without having to rely on expensive cosmetics. This chapter offers readers different ways to accesses this power by learning how to take care of our physical appearance and by taking control of their own aging process.

By now we all know the health benefits of keeping our bodies and minds active, eating well, and having a positive attitude toward ourselves. In this chapter, I take this argument a step further and connect it to our outer appearance: our skin, hair, teeth, clothing, and so on.

The same physical activities, the same nutrition and the same state of mind that gives us inner health and beauty also gives us outer beauty and keeps our skin, hair, and teeth healthy. For example, it is our brain that tells our skin to produce more or less oil or collagen. It's also our brain that signals our skin cell regeneration, which means that our state of mind directly affects our skin's condition. If we get angry, our faces turn red. If we get sad our faces drop. If we are happy, our faces glow. And if we don't get enough sleep, our skin becomes pale and lifeless. All this means that we have to think of our skincare in conjunction with our mental and physical health.

The condition of our skin says a great deal about how well we fit into and feel supported by our current environment. There is an unmistakable glow emanating from those of us who are happy and satisfied with our lives that no amount of cosmetic surgery can create. If for any reason we feel unsafe or not true to ourselves in our present environment, our skin may react developing blemishes, discoloration, dryness, and rashes. That's why many dermatologists recognize that some patients may need simultaneous treatment of their skin, mind, and emotion for best results.

Biology of Your Skin

Our skin consists of three layers: an outer layer called the epidermis, the middle layer called the dermis, and a fat layer beneath. The epidermis is the top layer of our skin, which acts as our body's shield against the outside world. Our main job is to keep our epidermis healthy and plump with proper nutrition, exercise, and skincare. The epidermis is the layer that we see when we look in the mirror. Although we all have this outer layer, its thickness differs from person to person. The epidermis protects us against bacterial, viral, and sun exposure. The outermost portion of the epidermis consists of dead cells. That's why sometimes after drying our face we may notice flaking skin on our forehead.

Sun can damage our epidermis, causing peeling, dryness, and wrinkles. With steady damage the wrinkles and lines will get deeper and more prominent. Sun is responsible for our premature aging. Those of us that were sun worshipers may show early signs of aging, including wrinkles and age spots. Wearing sunscreen at all times is one of the most important things that we can do for our skin's health. Ultraviolet light erodes our skin's support structure, breaks down our collagen (causing wrinkles), and penetrates deep into the underlying support structure of our skin. Sun damage is cumulative and irreversible.

Under our epidermis is our dermis, which acts as our skin's support. The epidermis and the dermis together make up our skin's essential defense system. The dermis consists of a single row of columnar cells in which young cells develop and move upward to the surface. All our facial cells are nourished the same way as the rest of our cells through proper nutrition. This is why what we eat or don't eat will show on our face. Our skin is a good indicator of our overall state of health.

The dermis contains the two essential proteins that keep our skin looking young, collagen and elastin. These two proteins give our skin its elasticity and flexibility. The dermis also holds our nerve receptors, blood vessels, and oils. Oils travel up our hair follicles to the skin's surface, where it forms a protective coat. The sweat and oil secretions from the dermal layer protect our skin from infections. By middle age we may have lost up to 25% of our collagen layer, and some of our oil glands tend to decrease their secretions. All these result in a greater tendency toward dryness.

Our dermis also contains layers of living tissues. These tissues are filled with elastin fibers that support our skin. As we age, some of these fibers break and our dermis is incapable of supporting our skin, resulting in lines and wrinkles. By our mid-fifties, the capacity for our skin to repair itself tends to slow down drastically. Remember, what happens in our dermis most often creates our facial aging. These effects are permanent. The only way to slow this process down is by maintaining our skin's health.

The deepest layer of our skin is made of fat cells and strands of connecting tissue. It functions as a kind of pillow, cushioning the internal organs, holding our body heat and giving contour to our skin. To keep it healthy, we need to drink plenty of water and avoid yo-yo dieting, which can deprive us of essential nutrients.

Premature aging of our skin is related to what are known as free radicals. Free radicals are produced by unprotected sun exposure, smoking, air pollutants, and stress. Over time our skin becomes stiff and discolored, loses its elasticity, and our levels of collagen and elastin break down, resulting in wrinkles. When our collagen breaks down, our skin sags and wrinkles. This process is accelerated by our exposure to free radicals.

By middle age we see clear evidence of this damage. For example, excessive exposure to ultraviolet radiation from the sun results in tissue inflammation that begins with free radical damage to skin cell membranes, followed by a release of harmful chemicals that damage collagen and elastin fibers. Our collagen and elastin fibers that were originally fluid and flexible become stiff and hard, resulting in our skin looking dry, saggy, and wrinkled.

A healthy approach to beauty is not to try pretending that our looks are not important, nor to take the other extreme by being obsessive about them. Rather, each one of us needs to take an honest assessment of the value that we place on beauty and determine how much money and time we are willing to spend on our appearance.

<u>Learn to Love the Skin You are In Today</u>

<u>Exercise I</u>

Assess your current feelings about your skin. Answer these questions honestly so you can recognize your likes and your dislikes about your skin.

1. What do you like about your skin? Why?
2. What don't you like about your skin? Why?

3. What are some concerns that you have about your skin?
4. What would you like to change about your skin?
5. What are some things that you would like to learn about taking care of your skin?
6. Do you believe that you are capable of learning and of implementing what you will learn?
7. Do you believe that with the changes that you are willing to make, you would feel better about your skin and your appearance?

By answering these questions, you become aware of all the things that you like as well as the things that you don't like about your skin and why you feel that way. Knowing how you feel about your skin today helps you devise your own individualized skincare plan that fits your lifestyle. Learning to accept the skin you are in means challenging your thinking by becoming less critical and judgmental. Continuing criticism, such as "I hate these wrinkles," "I look so old," and so on, will hinder your quest for a healthier you. So stop criticizing and start living.

Remember, beauty is feeling good about yourself with everything that you have and accepting it with pride. There is no single definition of beauty. Your beauty is a reflection of your overall quality of life.

In her book The Beauty Myth, Naomi Wolf describes the different attitudes women have toward aging. She writes "You could see the signs of female aging as diseased. Or you could see that if a women is healthy, she lives to grow old" (105).

What Does Your Skin Need?

Nutrition

Our brain, body, nervous system, skin, hair, nails, and teeth all need nourishment to stay healthy. They don't function well on fast foods, sugar, white flour, and fatty red meats. By now we are all familiar with the benefits of healthy eating. What we eat can accelerate or slow down our aging process. Nutritional deficiencies affect our skin, hair, nails, teeth, and our general health. Our skin is a mirror for what's going on inside our bodies. Bad nutritional choices as well as a poor lifestyle, such as smoking, inactivity, and persistent stress all contribute to poor blood circulation and the accumulation of free radicals.

Aging skin can be reversed by consuming large amounts of fruits, such as raspberries, blueberries and strawberries, all of which are powerful antioxidants. Fruits and vegetables provide us with the necessary substances called phytochemicals. This important substance keeps our cholesterol level normal, boosts our immune system, and reduces the effects of aging. For example, orange fruits and vegetables are rich in beta-carotene. Leafy greens are rich in Vitamin E, which helps protect our cell membranes and guards us against UV radiation. Foods such as almonds, sunflower, seeds, spinach, broccoli, olive oil, and flax seeds are all high in vitamin E. Yellow fruits are rich in vitamin C, which is involved in collagen production and protects our cells from free radical damage. All raw foods give our body the enzymes it needs to maintain good health, protect our skin's lipids, and supports collagen and elastin. They all protect our skin cells from environmental dangers.

Seeds, nuts, tofu, yogurts, chickpeas, lentils, flaxseed, and good proteins are important for our skin. They are necessary to form collagen, which is the major building block for our skin to repair itself. Good sources of proteins are fatty fish rich in Omega-3, chicken, turkey, legumes and beans. They help repair our skin just as any other organ in our body. As we age, our skin cells' turnover slows down. The best remedy for this is adequate protein intake so our skin's dermis receives enough amino acids to function well.

Another important food for our skin and hair are oils and complex carbs. Oils are found in olive oil, flax oil, nuts, seeds, avocado, almonds, and walnuts. The easiest way to reap the beauty benefits of these oils is to add them into our daily meals. Fatty acids and oils keep our skin moist, soft, and supple.

Complex carbs, such as brown rice, pasta, lentils, whole grains, barley, quinoa, squash, and pumpkins, are also very beneficial to our skin's health because they contain lots of fiber as well as an important antioxidant, selenium. Selenium is important in maintaining the youthfulness of our skin. Selenium can also be found in nuts, seeds, and seaweed.

Water is the best way to keep our skin hydrated. Water accounts for 70% of our skin's weight, so it makes sense that we need to continuously replenish fluids and keep our cells hydrated. Water helps our body flush away toxins, allows the smooth flow of nutrients into our cells, and keeps our organs functioning properly.

Add Fitness to Your Beauty Regime

What's good for our brain is good for our body, heart, and skin. Exercise improves blood flow to every organ in our body, so it makes sense that it would benefit our skin, which is the largest organ in our body. With exercise, we increase our circulation, which allows greater amounts of oxygen to be delivered to our skin cells, thereby helping our skin renew its cell production of collagen. Remember, any type of activity should be fun and enjoyable; otherwise it will not be continuous.

Sleep for a Beautiful You

A good night's sleep is important for our overall health. Lack of sleep depletes our energy. Our bodies send energy to our heart, intestines, and endocrine system before they send energy to our skin and hair. Poor circulation leads to sallow skin and dark circles under our eyes. The amount of sleep each of us needs varies from person to person, but the recommended time for adults is seven or eight hours of sleep each night. Sleep deprivation causes puffiness and wrinkles around the eyes, dark spots, dryness, blemishes, and sagging facial muscles. Reduced blood flow as a result of sleep deprivation causes our faces to look tired and wrinkled. Sleep is designed to restore us. It is during our sleep that our tissues are being repaired and our organs rest or flush out toxins. Sleep deprivation causes our brains to function poorly. Memory and concentration decline. Our facial muscles weaken, and our skin looks dull with blood-shot eyes. Aim for seven hours of sleep every night.

Good Skincare: Less is More

What is Your Skin Type?

Is your skin normal, oily, sensitive, or dry? Different skin types require different product formulations, but two important ingredients for every skin type are sunscreen and antioxidants. The key issue when it comes to your skin type is actually examining your skin's condition.

Test Your Skin Type

Clean your face, take a lens-cleaning tissue paper, and press it on different parts of your skin. If your skin is oily, the paper sticks and will pick up oily spots. If the paper does not stick to your skin, your skin is dry. If it sticks to your nose, forehead, and chin, but not to your cheeks, your skin is normal. But remember that your skin changes at different points throughout your life, so recheck your skin from time to time.

If you have dry skin, you need to use gentle nourishing oils which help you retain moisture in your skin. Moisture loss is definitely a symptom of dry skin, but simply giving the skin more moisture or drinking more water won't do the job. The problem might be that your skin does not have the ability to prevent water loss or to keep the right amount of water in your skin cells. The best beauty routine for dry skin is using a good moisturizer, using gentle cleansing products, exfoliating the outer layer to get rid of the unhealthy buildup of sun-damaged skin, using a humidifier, and applying a night cream with AHA or a BHA product.

If your skin is oily, it will shine. Oily skin must be kept clean and washed at least twice during the day and once in the evening. It's important to use an oil-free and water-based cleanser, as well as a toner or a clarifying lotion made for oily skin. Your moisturizer has to be water-based and oil free. Your goal with this type of skin is to control the oil, keep your pores from clogging, and retain your skin's natural oils.

If your skin is normal, use a water-based lotion and nondrying facial cleansers. Use a skin freshener for your skin and a moisturizer that is a lightweight soufflé type. Make sure that you drink eight glasses of water a day to flush your system of internal impurities and to restore the balance of water and oil on the surface of your skin.

If your skin is sensitive, it has less tolerance for chemical substances and reacts to bad eating habits, stress, hormonal changes, and environmental impurities. This type of skin tends to be more dry in certain areas of your face, and you may have frequent skin eruptions. It is important to meet your sensitive skin's needs with products that are tested to heal and relieve your skin conditions and to improve your skin's texture. Use products that are designed for sensitive skin. These products usually are gentle, oil-free and have water-holding agents to protect, condition, and smooth surface tissue.

Many times you might fall into the trap of thinking that if a product is expensive it's good for you. You need to realize that this is a trap that many women fall into. When it comes to beauty products, you have to become your own expert because no one else knows your skin and your lifestyle better than you do. You need to learn how to respond to your skin's needs and recognize that sometimes you need to be gentle or more proactive.

Your Skincare Regimen

As we age, our skin has different needs since it undergoes many alterations due to changes in our metabolism, wear and tear, diminished hormone production and oil secretion, poor diet, free radicals, lack of exercise, stress, and the use of harsh products that weaken our skin's protection barrier. Our skin becomes thinner, and it doesn't snap back as quickly as it used to.

Somewhere around our late forties or early fifties, we start noticing a few creases that won't go away. Our skin's cell turnover slows down, resulting in a duller looking skin. When dead cells pile up on the surface of our skin, our pores get clogged, resulting in more exaggerated wrinkles. The cumulative effects of free radicals also damage our skin cells and cause the breakdown of our collagen, which causes our skin to lose firmness. As we approach the menopause years and our skin gets thinner and drier, we need to use a slightly heavier moisturizer for our skin. Becoming aware of these normal changes to our skin's structure will help us create a regimen that fits our needs.

Four Basic Steps for Your Skincare

1. Cleanse your skin regularly.
2. Use a toner to close your pores after cleansing.
3. Renew your skin with an exfoliator twice a week.
4. Use a good mask once a week after steaming your face, and use a good moisturizer twice a day—once in the morning and once at evening.

Step One

Clean your face in the morning and evening because your skin comes into contact with dirt, make-up, and germs. Oil that is excreted from your skin attracts and holds dirt, causing your pores to clog. It's important to massage your cleanser into your skin to ensure your skin is clean. Massage your cleanser around your face in circular motions and rinse very well.

Cleansing is the most important facial beauty ritual. The secret to good cleansing is cleaning your face twice. The first time it will remove make-up and surface dirt. The second time gets deeper into the pores and removes dead skin cells. The best cleansing lotions are milky cleansing lotions or cleansing balms. If your skin is sensitive, stick to water-based, thin cleansing lotions.

Cleansers basically consist of oil and water. The oil dissolves the oil on your skin. Make sure that your cleanser is not too rich for your skin; otherwise it can clog your pores. If your skin is normal or dry, look for a milky or creamy cleanser. If your skin is oily, get an oil free cleanser, especially one with citrus to cut through the oil in your skin.

To apply, take a fingertip sized amount of your cleaner and massage it into your face and neck for about one minute. Then rinse it off with warm water to loosen clogged pores and to stimulate circulation. After you finish, repeat the same process the second time with the same cleanser, or you could use a smooth exfoliating cleanser. This time rinse it off with cold water to jazz up your circulation. This cleanser will penetrate deeper into your pores, giving you a healthier looking skin.

Step Two

Use a toner on your skin before you put on your moisturizer. Toners remove all traces of the cleanser and soften your skin. You can either buy a toner or you can make it at home. For example, you can mix one cup of peppermint tea with a cup of green tea. You can put it in a bottle with a spray top and keep it refrigerated for a refreshing mist. Or you can squeeze the juice from a chopped cucumber and rub it on your face. These home remedies work as well as store bought toners.

Step Three

Exfoliate your skin twice a week to rejuvenate it. Your skin undergoes a natural exfoliation process as new skin cells are produced in the bottom layer of your epidermis and old ones are shed. This rejuvenating process is intended to heal your skin. However, as you age this cellular process slows down, causing the buildup of dead skin cells. As you recall, the dermis is where collagen, elastin, and other proteins are made. As a result of aging, this layer weakens because of the loss of these proteins and your skin structure starts to collapse. That's when exfoliating comes in because it removes the dead layers of your skin. Make sure to gently massage your exfoliating cream into your face around your nose and chin. After you exfoliate, your skin will look and feel more refreshed.

You can make your own exfoliate with one tablespoon of sugar and one teaspoon of water. Mix the two together and rub the solution gently into your skin for about one minute. Then rinse with warm water. Your face will be left clean and refreshed.

Step Four

Moisturize your skin twice a day: in the morning and before you go to bed. Moisturizers keep your skin moist and well protected. When your skin is dry, even fine lines start to look like wrinkles. By adding moisturizer to your skin, you can temporarily plump it up, making it look more youthful. A good moisturizer protects your skin and slows down the evaporation of water, which helps your skin heal and recuperate by locking the skin's natural moisture inside. The most important function of your moisturizer is to maintain your skin's own protective barrier.

Younger skin has a stronger protective barrier because of the density of collagen fibers and better circulation in your skin. By middle age, your skin loses some of its protective strength as a result of pollution, poor diet, hormonal fluctuation, and water loss. Because of regular exposure to toxicities, proper moisturizing is a necessity. The best time to apply moisturizer is right after you wash or shower, when your skin is already damp and moist. Don't forget about your neck. Stroke upward, so you don't pull your skin down.

Moisturizers come in different forms. Cream forms are thicker and greasier. Lotions are lighter and more fluid. Gels are clear and the lightest of all. Remember one important fact: the thicker the texture, the more oil it contains—while the thinner the texture, the more water it contains. It's important to judge your moisturizer by its texture and understand what the texture tells you about its properties, helping you zero in on what you need for your skin type.

The most important ingredient in any good moisturizer is natural oils. Some of the best oils are olive oil and coconut oil. Moisturizers also need to have sun protection, SPF 15 or more. Remember to use a sunscreen which protects your skin against harmful ultraviolet rays that cause your skin to age. There are many moisturizers that have sunscreen protection included.

Sunscreens are important at any age, but especially for your aging skin. Ninety percent of your wrinkles are caused by the sun's ultraviolet (UV) light. This light, even at low level exposure, erodes your skin's support structure. It breaks down collagen causing wrinkles and sagging. Chronically exposed skin can develop a thick leathery texture because your body speeds up cell growth to thicken the top layer in a feeble attempt to block the UV light. If you choose to follow only one beauty tip in this book, remember to protect your skin from the sun.

At Home Facials

Some procedures are best left to professionals, but a relaxing mask applied in your home can make you feel fresher in just a few minutes. Apply a mask when your skin shows signs of stress or when you fell dehydrated. Depending on the ingredients, masks cleanse, tighten, exfoliate, or moisturize your skin.

You can make a homemade face mask quickly and easily. All you need is one egg yolk, honey, and olive oil. Whisk one egg yolk, and mix it with a teaspoon of honey. Mix well and then add one teaspoon of olive oil. Leave it on your face for ten minutes and then rinse it off. Your skin will be glowing.

Your Make-Up Routine

Less Is More

Let's start by demystifying the art of make-up and understanding that "less is more" at any age. Since many of us think that using make-up is complicated, I would like to bring forth the idea of simple make-up and a basic skincare routine. Our make-up at any age should be simple and natural so that people notice our faces and not our make-up. Make-up should be used to enhance our features, not hide them. The colors that we choose should harmonize with our complexion and skin tone so that they enhance our face, accentuate our best features, and hide some of the imperfections that come with age.

Make-Up Colors for Your Skin Tone

Even though this section emphasizes the importance of maintaining a harmonious look between your skin tone and your make-up colors, it's important to take it a step further by including your clothing. Creating an overall balanced look is important since your clothing is next to your face and it impacts the coloring of your face.

Light Coloring: You need to keep your foundation as close as you can to your natural tone. Do not try to wear a foundation that is a few shades darker than your skin tone. It will make you look older. Your eyes should be kept soft with light to medium color shades. Similarly for your cheeks, lighter coloring will be more flattering than deeper tones. Your lips should reflect your overall light look. Using pale color lip shades like peach, corals, or light rose will give you a more balanced look.

Clothing: Since your face is made up with light coloring, to balance you need to choose clothing that maintains a harmonious look. This means that light, delicate colors are going to balance your look. It's important to avoid dark colors that would overpower your look. For example, black would make you look older. The best alternatives could be taupe, brown, grey, or light navies.

Dark Coloring: Again, choosing a foundation that matches your skin tone is very important since your foundation covers your entire face. For your eyes, a dark mascara and an eye pencil to enhance your coloring will give you a youthful look. For a more natural look, you can use a brown eye pencil. For your eye shadow, you have a variety of strong colors to choose from. For your checks, the blush needs to have pigmentation and some depth. For your lips, you need to complement your strong look with a rich color lipstick. If you use a sheer natural-looking lipstick, then give more depth to your eye wear.

Clothing: Your wardrobe should include your favorite colors. For example, if you like black, you can wear it day and night. You need to make sure that your colors are vibrant and to stay away from light colors. White could only look good if you use colorful accessories and dramatic make-up.

Warm Coloring: You need to choose warm tones for your make-up to complement your look of golden or light red. You need to make sure that your foundation matches your skin tone because nothing can look worse than a darker foundation. Eyes are important to accentuate. A warm brown mascara will look better than black. Your cheeks should be kept warm with golden blush shapes in anything from salmon to bronze. Avoiding pink blushes is important because it will clash with your complexion. Your lip colors should have a warm base. For example, you could use a spice colored lip pencil, and a terracotta shade lipstick with a copper lip gloss. This look will compliment your warm complexion.

Clothing: Your clothing needs to compliment your warm tones near your face. You need to mix blacks, grey, and browns with warm colors. This look can also be achieved with accessories, scarves, and jewelry.

Clear Coloring: The key to this look is the contrast between your pale skin coloring and your dark hair. Foundation should match your complexion. Your eyes could stand out by using beautiful eye colors and a color pencil. Using an eyebrow pencil will also enhance your eyes and will give them a frame. Your blush should highlight your face. For example, a salmon color blush will look good. Or you could combine it with a bronzer. Your lips should be soft so as not to distract from your eyes. A cantaloupe color lipstick would look great.

Clothing: Your clothing should include bright colors, especially if you are only wearing one color. Avoiding earth tone colors is important because they will give you a washed out look.

Remember: Whatever coloring you have, the key to a youthful appearance is keeping your make-up simple and natural looking.

Your Aging Skin

As we age, our coloring changes, and many times we find that colors that looked good on us before no longer do. We need to be able to adjust our coloring to what looks good on us at our specific age. By our fifties our faces are going through major changes as a result of the changes in our muscles, the texture of our skin, and hormonal changes. But with good skincare, healthy nutrition, physical activity, good sleep, and good stress management techniques we can look good at any age.

As a general rule, the older we become the less make-up we need. Light natural shades for our eyes, lips, and cheeks will give us a more youthful look. By the time we get into our sixties, we need to start embracing the many signs on our faces that we have lived well. Our make-up should embrace these natural changes, so being understated is the magic of keeping a healthy and youthful glow.

It's time to part from the colors we have been wearing when we were younger. Choosing the right color is key. For example, if we develop a double chin, a little darker powder brushed along the jawline will help create the illusion of a firmer face. We need to choose the correct foundation since our skin starts to be noticeably thinner. To avoid drawing attention to any lines, it is important to apply natural shades on the face, eyes and lips to suit our changing color.

Make-Up Routine

Create Your Specific Look

A frequently asked question is "How do I create a simple everyday beauty routine?" A comprehensive make-up routine consists of six basic steps: foundation, concealer, powder, eye shadow, mascara, and lipstick. But you can create your individual look for day and night that expresses your taste and lifestyle. Don't be discouraged if you have not used make-up before. This is the time to learn. For example, you might prefer a natural look for day and a heavier look for the evening. Or you might prefer to use only a good moisturizer and a lip gloss in the daytime and add some eye shadow and blush for the evening. Remember, make-up is your own personal creation.

Foundation

Your foundation determines your entire look, because it can make you look ten years older or ten years younger. You should create a healthy, glowing look with a foundation that is light in texture and provides you with a natural look. If your skin is normal, then a sheer foundation is the best way to go especially for the day. Avoid a heavy looking foundation because it will make you look older and artificial looking.

Remember when you choose your foundation to make certain that the color matches your own natural skin tone. Your skin is the most important part of your make-up look, so making it appear youthful and natural is important. Foundation and powder (if you are using powder) are the basis of flawless looking skin, so try your best to choose the best one for your complexion and skin type. Your goal should be to look as if you're wearing no foundation at all.

Liquid foundation is the most popular, and it's suited for all skin types. It's available in every type of formula for every skin type, from oil-free, oil-absorbing formulas to moisturizing formulas for dry skin. Liquid foundation also comes in varying degrees of coverage, from sheer to medium. When applied, it provides more coverage than a tinted moisturizer but less than a cream or stick foundation.

Application

Foundation could be applied either using a sponge, a brush, or your fingers. Dip the sponge into your foundation and apply it all over your face, focusing on areas that need the most coverage. Blend it well, especially under your chin. For powder foundation, use a brush and swirl it around and then lightly apply it all over your face. Remember not to overdo the foundation.

Concealer

Concealers are your best friend since they function as a good cover for all the problem areas on your face. You can use a concealer to cover under-eye areas, breakouts, or broken capillaries. To cover under your eyes, the best choice is a creamy concealer because it's moist and easier to blend. But for breakouts you should use a much drier-textured concealer so it will adhere better and last longer.

Application

Use your ring finger to apply under-eye concealer. If you use a stick concealer, move from left to right. You can also use a stick concealer as a foundation for your eye shadow. Dab with your fingers a tiny amount of lightweight concealer next to the inner corner of your eye, and blend it downward toward your cheek by dabbing it gently with your finger away from your nose.

Face Powder (Optional)

Powders help set your make-up foundation as well as even your skin color. Your powder is the finishing step that helps your skin appear smooth and natural. Powders come in different forms. They come as loose, pressed, or compact. Try them out and decide which suits you best or whether you want to use powder at all.

Application

A cotton ball is used to apply loose or pressed powder. Remember not to use a lot of powder because it will create a cake effect on your face, which is not attractive, and it can also emphasize the lines on your face. A fluffy powder brush is an ideal tool to have for both the loose and the compact powders.

Blush and Bronzer

A blush gives you a youthful glow to your cheeks. Some blushes are more sheer while others contain heavier pigments, which will provide you with more coverage and color intensity. Use blush with moderation, especially during the day. The ideal application is only a hint of color. Rich colors and matte colors (no shine) are the best for daytime for all types of skins. Blushes come in cream form, gels, liquid, or powder. Powder blush is the most popular one because it's the easiest to control; therefore, it's offered in the widest range of shades. If you have light skin, go with a pale pink. If you have a medium skin tone, go with a coral or peachy. If your skin type is dark, go with a brownish orange color.

Bronzer

Bronzer is the secret to having an eternally youthful glow. Bronzers are available in many different textures and finishes. They come in powder form, cream form, or gel. Powder bronzer is the most popular type because it's easy to control and blend. It may be packaged in a compact or loose in a tub. Powder bronzer finishes range from matte to a heavy dose of shimmer. Sweep it across your face with a brush, and it will bring your skin to life. Cream bronzer works well on dry skin. It's perfect for days you don't want to wear foundation but you want just a little glow on your face. Gel bronzer works best on normal to dry skin and provides a much sheerer color than other bronzers.

Eyes

Eye Shadow

Eye make-up should accentuate both your natural eye color as well as the shape of your eyes. Eye shadow can add depth to your eyes or just bring them to life. It can also reshape your lids and make them look their best. When choosing eye shadows it's important to consider the texture and the finish. Both make a big difference in the effect they create and how dramatic they look. Too much color around your eyes can detract from your eye color. Soft colors found in your skin tone, such as vanillas, beiges, browns, and mauves are the best. Natural color shadows are easy to work with because they melt well with one another and complement most skin tones.

Eye shadows come in powder, cream, pencil, and liquid forms. Powder shadows come in matte to shimmer, iridescent to frosty, and in many different colors. Loose powder shadow is the easiest to blend, but you have to be a little more careful in the application because sometimes it falls off. This is not a big deal. After dipping your applicator in shadow, just make sure to tap the excess off before you apply it.

Cream shadows are also available in different finishes such as mattes and shimmers. These are a good option if you have dry lids. Pencil shadows are the most convenient to use because you can easily put them in a small purse and use them on the go. They are useful for the area close to your lash line because they are sharpened to a point and can be applied with precision. Liquid shadows usually come in a shiny, metallic finish and are the hardest to use because they don't blend well. Liquid shadow is used either as an eye liner or applied close to the lash line for a more intense look.

Application

Apply your base all over your eyes. Choose a neutral color from your eye shadow palette, and with a blender brush apply it all over your entire eye area. The base color will ensure that all additional colors will blend together. Apply a medium or darker color for your contour shade. Then apply a little darker color to give your eyes definition at the outer corners. Blend it all together to give an even look all over. Your mascara is next. Look straight ahead and brush your mascara with a clean brush along your lashes. If you want a heavier look, you can repeat twice.

Eyeliner (Optional)

Eyeliner is definitely an option, not a must, when you apply your make-up. Poorly applied eyeliner will make you look older, and your eyes will appear smaller. On the other hand, properly applied eyeliner opens your eyes. Eyeliner comes in pencil, liquid, cream, or gel. Whichever you choose to use, apply it with a light hand and make sure that you follow your entire eyelash line top and (if you want) bottom. Chocolate, brown, or charcoal are good colors because they are not as harsh as black. If you want a softer look, use an eye shadow as well. To draw a precise line, you need to hold your lid in place with your fingers. Remember, if your eyes are tired, using an eyeliner will draw more attention to them.

Eyebrows

Let's not forget about your eyebrows since they are a major part of your face. Unkempt eyebrows make your look older. Good eyebrows have a classic, well-groomed shape, and they lift up your entire face. As you age, your eyebrows naturally become thinner due to tweezing, waxing, and the weakening of your hair follicles. Make sure that you groom your brows at least once a week. You can use tweezers or wax and do it yourself or have a professional do it for you. If you are tweezing, tweeze after you shower because your skin will be softer, so your hair will come out easier. Always pull your brows in the direction of your hair growth.

Application

Make sure to buy a good pair of tweezers with a pointed tip. Always pluck below your brow line so your hair will grow back in the same line. Use the top of your brow to guide you on how to shape your bottom ones. If your brows are sparse, fill them in taking an angled brush and pressing a little eye shadow to your brow, or fill them in with the same color pencil as your brows.

Mascara

Mascara is the most important element of your make-up routine because of the definition it creates. Full, thick lashes open up your eyes and make them look more alive. Mascara comes in multiple formulas that give you a variety of results. You have thickening mascara, lengthening mascara, waterproof mascara, curling mascara, and defining mascara. Choose the formula that can help you achieve the look you want.

Application

You need to make sure that the brush is clean to avoid clumping or smudging. Apply upward from lower to upper lashes. Start from the middle and then move to the outer edges. If you give a few coats, it will create a thicker look. If you want to give your eyes a more open look, you may want to use an eyelash curler before you apply your mascara. It will give your eyes an open look as well as lift the look of your eye make-up.

Lipstick

Some lipsticks have more coverage and moisture, while others might just give you a sheer wash of color that looks and feels like it's not there. You will find many textures of lipstick in a big variety of finishes and colors. Play, test, and try a bunch until you find what you want in a lipstick or lip gloss. Keep in mind that keeping your lips moist is always very important.

Lipstick is composed of pigment which determines the color. A good color lipstick can make you look alive or pale. For example, a sheer lipstick will give you an understated look with a hint of color and shine. Cream lipsticks are also known as moisturizing lipsticks. They have a velvety texture, and they keep your lips moist. Matte lipsticks last longer because they contain the most pigment. They provide deep color with a flat look. Frosted lipsticks are also heavy pigment colors with an iridescent coverage. Lip glosses will give you a clear, shiny look. They are usually worn over lipstick to give a sheer look.

For daytime, you can go for a sheer or a light lipstick. Use a lip liner first to give your lips a nice shape, and then apply it all over your lips. Your lipstick will last longer and will not smudge. For evening, you can add a little more depth to the colors you are already using. For example, you can add a darker eye shadow to get a more dramatic look. You can apply black mascara to your upper and lower lashes. Or you can use a darker lip color and then add a little lip gloss for a shinier look.

Application

First outline your lips with a sharp pencil, and then fill in the rest of your lips to give color and depth to your lipstick or gloss. Then apply your lipstick, followed by your lip gloss on top for a moist effect. Use nude for a light shade lipstick and a darker color for any other lipstick color. Remember, your lips will look softer if you don't use a lip liner. As you age, you look better with a creamy lipstick rather than a matte because it will give you more shine and moisture.

Remember, whatever you choose, make-up should be fun and easy to use. Nora Ephron in her book, *I Feel Bad About My Neck*, talks about maintaining her skin. "Maintenance takes up so much of my life... You know what maintenance is, I'm sure. Maintenance is what we mean when we say, after a certain point it's just patch, patch, patch. These patches are the difference between a fifty-year-old woman who looks forty, and a fifty-year-old woman who looks sixty. The truth is that we cannot let ourselves go."

Make-Up Tools

There are a few essential tools which you need for your make-up routine:

1. Face cloths to wash your face
2. Soft facial tissues
3. Cotton balls

Brushes should be made of gentle natural fibers. For the brushes to work well, their bristle cannot be too soft because they won't be able to pick up and put down color. But they cannot be too hard because that will cause irritation to your skin. The few essential brushes you should have on hand are a powder brush, eye shadow brush, and a lip brush. Remember to clean all your brushes regularly to give you the best application and clarity of color. Also, wash your hands every time you touch your face.

Your make-up can be understated or overdone. As you get older, your make-up should be natural and convey to the world that you feel good and secure about yourself. Keeping make-up simple eliminates the artificial look and emphasizes your unique features. Ultimately, what you want is for your make-up to enhance your look and keep you looking as young and as natural as possible.

Perfumes

We are all different individuals, but we all want to look good, feel good, and smell good. Smelling good is about pleasing our senses. Perfumes reveal our personality, our taste, and even our mood. Choosing the right perfume could be hard because there so many to choose from. The easiest way to buy a perfume is by testing it on our body. Apply it to your wrist, wait a few seconds for it to evaporate, and then sniff it. If the smell pleases you, then it's a good choice. But if there is a slightest tinge of uncomfortable odor, we should move on to the next one.

When we buy a perfume, we need to consider our body's chemistry. What smells good on our friend and seems just right may not produce the same effect on us. Fragrance develops differently on individual skin types, depending on natural skin oils, body temperature, and the season. If our skin is oily and it's summer, perfume will evaporate faster; so we might need a stronger scent. If we have dry skin, the fragrance will sink into our skin; so we might have to apply the perfume more than once to keep the scent potent.

Fragrances come in different categories. Floral is a blend of flowers. Oriental scents are mysterious and exotic. Spicy scents include extracts of vanilla, ginger, cinnamon, and cloves. Finally, fruity fragrances are a blend of lemon, lime, and mandarin.

Body Skincare

Just as our faces need care, so does the rest of our body. Our bodies get wrinkled, sunburned, and spotty exactly as our faces do. So the question remains, how do we keep our bodies youthful and glowing? The simple fact is that what works for our faces works for our bodies as well. Every aspect of our skincare designed to work from our neck up will work fine from our neck down. The names of the products may differ, but when it comes to the health and appearance of our skin, it's always about the best results. Skin is skin from head to toe.

Your Body's Skincare Routine: Clean, Exfoliate and Moisturize

Clean by using a good body wash. Body washes use the same detergent-based cleansing agents as your hair shampoos. They tend to be less dry then bar soaps and cause less dryness to your skin.

Exfoliate by using a good body scrub to remove your dead cells. Body brushing is all your skin needs. Removing your dead skin body cells makes it easier for your skin to absorb the moisturizer and keep your skin looking healthy. One of the most affordable tools is a loofah. It's used to remove dead skin cells that clog your pores and keeps your skin dry. Work it in circular movements to help stimulate your circulation. Exfoliating once a week will give your skin a healthy glow.

Moisturize to keep your skin moist. If you have dry skin, you need a rich textured moisturizer containing oils to keep your skin moist. The smoother your skin, the healthier it looks. If your skin is oily, you need to use a lighter textured lotion that is oil free. The best time to moisturize your skin is after a shower because the moisturizer penetrates better into your skin. Once you have gently patted yourself dry with a towel, you should coat your body with oil or lotion by applying your moisturizer in gentle strokes aiming upward from bottom to top of your body.

Remember that your skin's dryness is affected by the air around you. Dry air sucks the moisture out of your skin so it feels dry. Using an air humidifier is strongly recommended. You could also place a bowl of water near a source of heat and add a few drops of essential oils. The vapors will keep the air moist, so your skin can absorb the moisturizer better and keep your skin moist and healthy looking.

Your hands get as much exposure in daily life as your face. Many of us never pay attention to our hands even though they are such an important part of our appearance. Your hands get dry, rough, cracked, and wrinkled. Using a good hand cream and getting a manicure once a week could alleviate some of these problems. Your nails are very porous and can become dehydrated just as easily as your skin. So it's not surprising that oil is your nails' best friend. You can use any vegetable oils and massage your nails every day before bedtime to enhance circulation.

You have a choice when it comes to your nails. Do you want to bring attention to them or deflect attention? For example, if you want the deflect attention from your hands, having short nails and a light nail polish is the perfect look. Soft-color nail polishes will not be so visible as dark nail polishes, and your hands will not stand out as much. Keeping your nails short, clean, and neat while using a natural color for the polish will deflect attention from your hands. Whenever you can, wear gloves to protect your hands and nails from dryness, discoloration, and wrinkles, and use a hand moisturizer every day to keep your hands soft and healthy looking.

Get a manicure once a week, or just change the nail polish to give your nails a fresh look.

Home Manicure

1. Remove your existing nail polish with a nail polish remover.
2. Gently file your nails to the shape that you want.
3. Soften the cuticles around your nail if you are planning to cut them. You can soak your nails in warm water to help soften them.
4. Moisturize your hands and cuticles with a good hand cream. Wash down the moisturizer to clean your nails.
5. Apply nail polish in two coats to last longer. Then put on a top coat to add shine.

Remember that it's important to allow enough time for the polish to dry.

Your feet need attention as well. How much attention do you pay to your feet? Most of us pay little attention to our feet in spite of the torture we inflict upon them with tied shoes, high heels, and the walking and standing that they endure. We can neglect our feet for only so long before they fight back and leave us bunions, corns, and calluses.

To take care of your feet, soak them in warm water, exfoliate and massage with a good cream to keep them moist, soft, and healthy. You can give yourself a pedicure or have it done at a salon every few weeks. Whatever style pedicure you choose, you should cover the basics: soak your feet in warm water for about ten minutes; exfoliate with a good foot scrub; and moisturize with a good moisturizing cream. It's important to take your time and massage the cream all over your feet and between your toes.

Beautify Your Teeth

Don't let your teeth give your age away. Your lips dramatically outline your mouth; therefore, your teeth must not detract from your face. Your lips, teeth and smile make your face radiate or not. Your teeth are the center of every moment of your days. Taking good care of them should be part of your make-up routine.

Every time you open your mouth to speak, smile, eat, or cry, your teeth are fully exposed. The life that you are living is reflected in your teeth. Your tooth enamel is porous, so teeth get easily stained from coffee, tea, wine, fruits and all types of foods that you eat. So keeping your teeth clean is very important for appearance as well as health. There is nothing more aesthetically appealing than a healthy set of bright teeth.

Maintenance

Maintain your teeth and gums by brushing and flossing them at least twice a day or after every meal. When you don't brush your teeth after a meal, you are inviting all the stain-producing foods to get cozy on your enamel and settle in for the next eight hours, or until you brush your teeth. It's important to use a soft toothbrush to protect your teeth from irritation as well as to protect your enamel. Hard toothbrushes are too abrasive and can easily erode your enamel. Change your toothbrush every three to four months to maintain healthy teeth. An important maintenance strategy for your teeth is flossing to remove the gunk between your teeth and gums, staving off gum recession. Using a good mouthwash twice a day will help you keep your teeth and breath clean and fresh.

If your teeth are persistently yellow and stained, you can use a teeth-whitening solution. There are many different options and brands. It does not have to be expensive to work. Try out a few types, and find out which works best for your teeth. Don't forget to visit your dentist twice a year for a cleaning and check-up to keep your teeth healthy.

Nothing ages you more and spoils your appearance as much as your teeth. Gray teeth, yellow teeth, strained, or broken teeth make you look older. What's nicer than flashing a set of healthy white teeth every time you smile? It's a strong message that you are sending, which says you are healthy, vital, and confident in your appearance. After you spend time and money improving your make-up, you don't want a mouthful of yellow teeth. Teeth are an important part of your appearance that should not be neglected.

Healthy Hair

Another important feature that frames our faces is our hair. Our hair has an enormous power over our state of mind because it makes us look and feel good or bad about ourselves. Our hair makes a strong statement about our individuality. Yet, if we stop for a moment and consider the abuse that our hair takes with blow drying, coloring, curling, twisting, and pulling, it is no wonder that many times our hair just gives up. When our hair looks good, we feel great, but when our hair looks bad, we feel down and depressed. So the big question is, "What does our hair need to stay healthy, and how do we accomplish this important task?"

The real job of our hair is to protect our head against heat loss and against the potentially harmful rays of the sun. If we examine our hair's anatomy, we discover that our hair emerges from the follicle which is below the surface of our scalp. We have on the average 100,000 follicles. The more dense our follicles, the more hair we will have. Each follicle controls the hair growth out of it. Both our hair and our follicles repeatedly die and regenerate throughout our life span.

At the base of our follicles is the part of the hair called the roots. Tiny blood vessels at the base of our follicles feed our hair nutrients to support our hair growth, which means that what we eat affects the health and growth of our hair. Healthy hair growth needs the same type of nutrients, foods, vitamins, minerals and proteins, as the rest of our body.

Our hair grows out of follicles, and within a few days they become visible. By the time our hair becomes visible, it's actually nonliving tissue composed of dead keratin cells. These keratin cells are woven together like a tiny rope to form our hair strand. Each strand has three layers: the outer layer called the cuticle, which protects our hair against water loss; the cortex, which gives our hair strength; and the medulla, which reflects light and gives our hair sheen and tone.

Our hair does not grow every day; rather, it goes through phases of growth and rest. The active growth phase allows new hair to grow. In the resting phase, our hair does not grow. Under normal circumstances our hair growth follows this pattern of rest and activity. But sometimes these cycles are disrupted and we begin to lose hair. There are many reasons for hair loss. One is genetics. The gene for hair loss can be inherited from either our mother or father. Others factor could be hormonal changes (like those during pregnancy or menopause), nutrition, stress, lack of activity, depression, and age. For example, a shortage of iron in our diet could cause hair loss. It's important to find out what the causes of our hair loss are and take steps to correct them.

Most of the time, hair loss develops slowly over many years, and eventually we begin to see scalp and not hair. We tend to get an oval area of baldness on top of our head and a thinning of our hair around our hairline. But most of us lose as much as 50% in the affected area of our head before we start noticing hair loss. Often this hair loss is only temporary, like during pregnancy, after which it goes back to its normal rate of shedding.

Help is not easy to get because lost hair very rarely comes back. The only recommended F.D.A. treatment is Minoxidil, also known as Rogaine. Minoxidil comes in two strengths. One is 2% concentration used by women, and the other is 5% concentration used by men. Usually, you can see results after six month of usage. Minoxidil, however, does not work for everyone. To maintain its full benefits, we should continue using it indefinitely.

Your Hair Care Routine

Similar to your skin, your hair and scalp need to be kept clean. If your scalp is dirty, it clogs your pores, causing unhealthy looking hair as well as hair loss.

Steps to Take for Healthy Hair

Shampoos and Conditioners

First, you need to find a good shampoo and conditioner for your hair. Shampoos are labeled for different types of hair such as dry hair, oily hair, and normal hair. Find the right shampoo for you.

Conditioners are important. They bind to your hair making it stronger, softer and more resilient. It protects your hair against damage due to brushing, blow drying, and straightening.

Root lifters coat each individual hair fiber, swell your cuticles, and double their width. Your hair will look fuller as a result.

Hair Color

Before you start thinking about coloring your hair, you need to ask yourself: "What would I like to change about my hair? Is it the color, the style, or both? Do I want to brighten my original hair color? Or do I want to make a drastic change in my hair color?" Knowing the answers to these questions is important before you start playing with your hair color. You can also consult a hair colorist at a beauty salon. Once you have all the information you need, you can choose to have it professionally done or do it yourself.

There are many different types of hair colors, but the most popular is permanent color. Permanent color can change your look from brown to blond or vice versa. It can also cover your gray hair without altering your natural hair color. Permanent colors last for approximately two months, or until your next cut.

It's important to acknowledge that any type of color you use has chemicals that can damage your hair. These chemicals (i.e. ammonia and peroxide) can cause frizziness and dryness, split ends, and sometimes even hair loss. Some brands have less chemicals and more protection built into them. It's important to become an educated consumer. For example, henna, the oldest way to color hair, is 100% natural and by far the gentlest. There are three types of henna: red, neutral, and black.

Another way to change your looks is by adding some highlights, which is a less invasive process. Highlighting brightens your hair by adding light to it. It could be one shade lighter than your natural hair color or a few shades lighter. As you age, lightening your hair gives you a brighter look.

If you are only trying to cover up gray roots, the best solution is matching the coloring to your natural hair color as much as possible. If your natural color is a warm tone, that means you need to look for a warm color shade with golden undertones.

Colored hair needs special care to look healthy and shiny. On the market today there are many different shampoos and conditioners for colored hair. If you are applying two processes to your hair, such as a color and perm or a relaxer, you need to wait at least two weeks between each process. Never do them on the same day.

Haircuts

No matter what kind of haircut you choose, if it's a good cut your hair will move well, it will be easy to maintain, and it will look good from every angle. A good cut accentuates your good facial features and plays down your unattractive ones. For example, it could accentuate your eyes or your cheek bones and hide some of your wrinkles or brown spots under your eyes.

Your hair cut—whether short, layered, or long—decorates your face and body and serves as an intimate expression of who you are. In other words, a haircut not only has to suit your face and body, but your personality and lifestyle as well. Experimenting with different trends in hairstyles is fun, and it will definitely refresh your look. But remember that a bad haircut can make you look older, no matter how young you are.

Your Facial Structure

Before you get a haircut, familiarize yourself with your facial structure. Here are a few suggestions that hairstylists agree on. If your face is round with a wide chin, you would look the best in a cut where your face appears longer. A short cut with layers on the top for height, tapered around your ears, will elongate your face. Do not make your face look wider by having extra width on the sides. If your face is oval with a prominent jawline and long chin, you need a cut that will widen your narrow face. Going for a short or chin length layered cut, full at the sides and tapered in, is the best cut for you. This cut will de-emphasize the length of your oval face. You can also add some bangs, which will frame your face. If you have high chin bones or a delicate and pointy chin, you will look good with a longer haircut. Avoid very short cuts. You can have some soft bangs and short layers on top. Long hair on your neck that is wispy at the bottom will help emphasize your bone structure.

Your Hair Texture

Your hair's texture plays an important role in your haircut as well. If your hair is fine and thin, the trick is for the cut to make it look fuller. You can accomplish this with a slightly layered cut, which will add more volume to your hair. Layers on top of your hair will lift it, and, as a result, your hair will look fuller and thicker. For styling your hair, you should use a thickening spray, but avoid heavy gels because they will make your hair sticky.

If your hair is curly, you can have it cut to any length, but adding some layers will keep locks from looking like a bush. Find a stylist that has the skill to cut this type of hair. It's important to cut your hair wet because it's easier to see its natural shape. Curly hair is about movement and not messiness, which is why a good layered cut will work well with your hair's natural shape.

If your hair is straight, the best cuts are either a blunt cut like a pageboy's or a bob cut slightly layered. For an edgier look, try thick, blunt, fringy bangs, sides tapered into points, and a slightly graduated back. These types of cuts will give your hair movement and some swing. You can also go with a short razor cut with tapered sides and longish spikes or a slick straight hair style. When styling your hair, direct air flow down the hair shaft to emphasize surface shine.

Wavy hair needs enough length to fall into its natural pattern. Your best results would be cutting it in long enough layers so that it's shaped where your natural wave falls. If you cut it too short, you can lose the wave or it can became frizzy and difficult to manage.

Remember that styling products are essential for all types of haircuts, and so are a good brush and blow dryer. For long hair a square-shaped, natural bristle brush is best because the spaced out bristles are gentle on your hair. A round brush will give you a smoother, more polished look. It curls the ends of your hair, which adds volume. Round brushes are great for styling straight hair. A midsized brush is good for shoulder length or shorter hair, and a large brush is best for longer hair. Make sure that your blow dryer has a diffuser attached to it because it protects your hair against extensive heat damage, and it gives your hair more body and volume.

Hair Problems

Dry hair needs more moisturizer. The best treatment is to steam your hair in a warm shower and use a good conditioner and shampoo for dry hair. Don't over process your hair with too frequent coloring, perms, or relaxers. Any process is bad for your hair and makes it drier. If your hair has no volume, use a very light conditioner. Use a good clarifying shampoo and a good root-lifter product. Frizzy hair needs to be treated gently. Use a good conditioner, and leave it on your hair for one minute before washing it off. Don't wash your hair every day because you rob it of the natural oils that help your hair stay in place. Finally, split ends are easy to deal with: just cut them off.

If there is one lesson to learn from reading this chapter, it's that we are fully responsible for our outer beauty. We need to move away from our mind-set that has kept us inactive or reliant on outside sources to make decisions for us. We need to take charge of our looks and wellbeing by eating well, exercising, getting enough sleep, learning to relax, drinking enough water, and developing a positive mind-set toward aging. Let's use the knowledge that we have acquired through reading this book, as well as our common sense, to guide us on this important journey to self-discovery.

CHAPTER VIII

The Psychology of Dressing

> "The fashionable woman wears clothes. The clothes don't wear her."
>
> Mary Quant

How does a fifty or sixty-year-old woman dress? Exactly her age, not young, not old? Does she hold on to her clothing because it's part of her history or because she is afraid of change? Is she confused about her appearance? Is she conflicted about what's appropriate to wear at her age? Should dressing be age appropriate? And if yes, then where are these messages coming from? Does our culture imposes restrictions on our dressing and self-grooming? Do we hear messages that tell us that certain styles and colors are not appropriate after a certain age? These are some of the questions my generation of women faces, which cause us confusion, anxiety, and unnecessary stress.

Our culture gives us conflicting messages about our clothing. On the one hand, in movies, magazines, and ads we see women our age dressed like teenagers. On the other hand, our society instills in us an "age-appropriate" dressing style. So which is it? Having recently turned sixty-eight myself, I have decided to tackle some of these questions and redefine what today's fifty or sixty-year-old woman looks and dresses like. If dressing is a personal expression of our personality and creativity, which I strongly believe it is, then how can any restrictions be put on it? How can our freedom of expression be denied? How can our creativity be restricted at middle age or beyond? And if we are still haunted by the old rules that governed many generations of women before us, then our time has arrived to re-examine those old rules and decide what works today.

I started answering some of these questions for myself many years ago. Since I was always free spirited, creative, and an independent thinker, especially when it came to fashion, I was able to create my own personalized dressing style. My clothing always reflected my unique personality and love of fashion. I had never followed any fashion trends. I never wanted to look like anyone else. I followed my heart, and dressing become a labor of love that persists to this day. My clothing clearly reflects who I am and how I feel about myself. My age is never a factor when I choose a piece of clothing.

So, with this in mind, I decided to open an honest dialogue between our cultural messages, our psychology of dressing, and middle age. I was determined to clarify some of the confusions and insecurities that my generation of women are facing at this juncture in their lives. I strongly maintain that there is no such a thing as age-appropriate dress, since our clothing reflects our individual styles, creativities, lifestyles, evolving personalities, tastes, needs, likes, and dislikes.

To take this argument a step further: if what I am proposing is true, that there is no age appropriate dressing, then what? What exists today is our individual free expression, which incorporates everything that we are, including our lifestyle, interests, values, beliefs, habits, and the environment that we live in. Just as our inner self reflects this reality, so does our outer self, including our grooming, self-care, and psychology of dressing.

Our generation of women, baby boomers, look younger and more physically and mentally fit than previous generations of women. We put physical fitness on the map. More and more women in their sixties, seventies, and even eighties work out at the gym or in their homes. They are better informed about the health benefits of keeping active, eating properly, getting proper sleep, de-stressing, and maintaining a balanced lifestyle. So it makes sense that our clothing should reflect this newfound freedom, wisdom, and strength that we now possess.

A woman in her fifties or early sixties is not old, but neither is she young. We are somewhere past the middle of our lifecycle, which means that a big part of our lives is still ahead of us. We need to start paying attention to the second part of our lives and equip ourselves with the knowledge necessary to look and feel good about ourselves and our appearance.

Our language of fashion is expressed by the way we feel about ourselves and how we present ourselves to the world. Fashion is our instant language. It reflects our personality, our feelings, our creativity, our self-esteem, and our level of confidence. Our clothing is a clear reflection of our persona and our overall lifestyle. When it comes to our clothing, there are no rules because we are all individually different, with different needs, tastes, body shapes, and lifestyles. This means that our psychology of dressing is a true reflection of who we are at this junction of our lives.

If we accept our flaws and optimize our positive qualities, we will radiate a sense of self- worth that is the cornerstone of having a great style. On the other hand, if we are critical of our looks, our clothing will clearly reflect that reality. We all have flaws, but once we accept them and work with them we can start focusing on what makes us look good. By accomplishing this important task, we take ownership of our bodies and minds. It might take a complete change in our overall psychology of dressing to achieve this important outcome.

There is no stronger evidence of the interconnection that exists between our minds and bodies than in our psychology of dressing. The psychology of dressing simply means that the way we dress is the way we feel. If we feel good or bad about ourselves and our bodies, this feeling will be reflected in our clothing and our general self-grooming. One major question emerges from these considerations. Are we what we look like? Or is our self-grooming a clear reflection of how we feel at a certain moment of time? If there is a disconnect between our style of dress and our personality, we might feel ungrounded and off balance, which could cause dissatisfaction with our looks. That's why it's important to create a balance between our personality and our style of dressing, which is the main focus of this chapter.

Many times we wonder why certain people dress the way they do. Why are their clothes too big or too small? Why are they wearing those colors against their faces? Why are they so overmatched? Why do they wear such outdated outfits? Why do they dress like their daughters? One reason could be that their clothing reflects their sense of insecurity. They may feel uncomfortable with their bodies, or they may have some unresolved inner conflict that they have a hard time expressing. Or maybe it's simple lack of awareness of what looks good on them. All this means that our clothing is an extension of who we are, how we feel, and how connected or disconnected we are from our self.

When we shop, we consider consciously or unconsciously our dress size, color, age, fit, culture, and lifestyle. We either work to incorporate all these aspects into our style of clothing or we go against them. Our closets are a true reflection of this reality.

We all try to express or hide something with the clothing that we are wearing. But how many of us are aware of this simple fact or realize its deep meaning? For example, if our closets are filled with baggy, shapeless pieces, it might mean that we are trying to hide our body. Or if our closets are full with overly youthful pieces, it might mean that we are afraid of getting old, and we might dress the way we dressed thirty years ago. Or, if our closets are filled with old pieces that don't fit us, it might mean that we pay no attention to our self-grooming. Simply examining the content of our closets will help us understand our psychology of dressing since our closets are a clear reflection of our true fashion style.

Examine Your Closet

Exercise I

Open your closet and go through its contents. Familiarize yourself with the types of clothing that you have, and think about the message you are sending to yourself and to the outside world about yourself.

1. What does your closet say about you?
2. Does it reflect the person that you are today?
3. Can you identify any reasons for choosing your wardrobe?
4. Is your closet full of pieces that you never wear?
5. Do you often feel that you have nothing to wear even though your closet is full?
6. Do you like the things that you see?
7. What do you like and what don't you like? Make a list and describe why you feel that way.

If you are satisfied with your answers about your wardrobe, keep on doing what you are doing. But if you are unhappy with the content of your closet, keep reading.

Creating a wardrobe that reflects your present lifestyle is not an easy task since you have to familiarize yourselves with your taste in clothing, your body shape, the changes that you are willing to make, your career, your social life, your interests, and your feelings about yourself.

But in order to be able to accomplish this important task, you need to examine your inner self, including your self-confidence, your emotions, and your feelings about your body image. Only after you have carefully examined these areas of your life can you start addressing your outside appearance, including your clothing, accessories, make-up and self-grooming. Without both, the changes are incomplete and of short duration. The strong interconnection between your inner and outer self cannot be avoided. If there is a disconnect between the two, nothing will feel right and you will short change your quality of life.

Your History of Dressing

Our history of dressing started early in our childhood years when we internalized messages passed down by important figures in our lives. One example could have been our mother's dressing style or the style of any other significant adult that made an impression on our lives. Getting in touch with those early influences can help us better understand our present-day psychology of dress and move on, if that style of dress no longer feels right.

Exercise II

The following questions will help you get you in touch with your history of shopping and the major influences surrounding your dressing behavior.

1. Who taught you how to dress?
2. How did that person dress?
3. What did you learn about dressing?
4. At what age did you start dressing yourself?
5. Did your style change throughout the years? How?
6. What were the major triggers for your changes?
7. Were you aware of them at the time?
8. What are the things that stayed the same?
9. How would you describe your style today?
10. Do you enjoy getting dressed? Why?
11. Do you wear the same outfits every day, or do you like to wear something different each day?
12. What would you like to change about your wardrobe?
13. Are you ready to implement those changes right now?

If your answer to the last question is yes, then your job has just begun. These questions help you identify where you learned how to dress and the impact that it had on your dressing psychology. For example, if you buy more then you need, never wear some of the pieces that you buy, or don't throw out the pieces that you don't like, it might mean that you have internalized these types of shopping behaviors from someone significant in your life. Examining your shopping behavior and understanding that your early experiences had a strong impact on many areas of your life, including your style of dress, is important for being able to move forward.

Early in our lives, we internalize different messages about shopping, dressing, and self-grooming from significant people from our environment. We have learned these messages and use them automatically all our lives. If we are not consciously aware of them, we can become stuck with them even if they don't work well for us. One of these impediments could be emotional shopping. In the chapter on nutrition, I talk about emotional eating filling a void, an emptiness in our lives. Now I will focus on emotional shopping since there are lots of similarities between the two.

Emotional shoppers use shopping as self-medication. When they are upset, bored, angry, depressed, or lonely they could reward themselves by going shopping. It could also be a sign of their insecurity or competitiveness. Whatever the reasons are, they feel good for the moment, but once they get home and start unpacking, they might feel a sense of guilt. Many women call shopping their best form of therapy since the feel good chemical dopamine is activated, and it makes them come back for more and more.

If shopping is our form of self-soothing, then our association between shopping and relieving our discomfort will strengthen over time, and we could become compulsive shoppers. Stores reinforce these types of shopping behavior because they are attractive and addictive. For example, when we walk into a store, we can try on everything and no one disturbs us. It gives us something to do and something to focus our attention on. There is nothing wrong with buying clothing to make ourselves feel good. If anyone believes in the power of dressing well, it's certainly me, but there is something wrong when a piece of clothing replaces our expression of true emotions or blocks our path to a healthy resolution.

To get rid of emotional shopping, we need to identify our shopping patterns as well as our triggers. We need to ask ourselves, "Why we are buying these outfits? Are they necessary or are they just mindless purchases?" Once we identify our triggers for compulsive shopping, we can move on and start making small changes in our shopping behavior.

The other extreme of compulsive shoppers are those who find shopping stressful and boring. Every time this type of person walks into a store, they feel like running out. For them shopping is a stressful event and a chore that they could do without. They always complain that they have nothing to wear, but they do nothing about it because for them shopping is anxiety-provoking and a routine governed by old rules.

Another impediment to our shopping behavior could be living by the old rules that governed many previous generations of women. The old-fashioned rules established forty or fifty years ago still govern some of our lives even though fashion has evolved from when women dressed according to their age, when things were overmatched, when we stopped wearing whites in the fall, when we wore black mainly for the winter months, when we did not mix colors or patterns together, when we wore the same color shoes and bags and so on. All those rules do not apply today, since almost everything goes together. We just have to learn how to coordinate our outfits in a harmonious way.

But the biggest influence on our shopping behavior is our age. As we get closer to middle age, acknowledging our age or our process of aging can be hard to face. This fact is many times reflected in our clothing style. For example, some of us dress older then we are, or younger, or never change our style of clothing. We wear the same size, color, shape and type of clothing for many years. The only way to keep the same look for years is to trap ourselves in a time warp. If we dress older than we are, we are avoiding examining our aging process by not acknowledging where we currently are. If we dress more like our daughters, we are making an attempt to hide our age, which at times might draw negative attention to ourselves. So the question is, "How do we find a balance between the person that we are and our outer appearance?"

Many times we equate aging with loss of beauty and vitality. We start thinking about what is appropriate to wear for our age. Adjusting our style to fit a particular age, if there is such a thing, is a mistake. Staying away from particular colors or styles is very restrictive and unnatural. Feeling comfortable and confident about our looks is the only thing that counts at any age, but especially middle age. We need to find the right balance between what looks good on us, our personality, and our lifestyle. Let's not stop our growth; instead, let's allow our fashion style to evolve.

Your Psychology of Dressing

There are four basic factors that determine if your outfit is flattering or not: **fit**, **shape**, **color**, and **fabric**.

Fit is important because the right fit can make you look slimmer than you actually are. For example, if something is too big or too small, you can look ten pounds heavier. If something is too big, you get lost in it, and if something is too small, it's tight and it might show your bulges. A good fit is the essential piece of your clothing style puzzle. How clothes hang on your frame and hug your curves makes a big difference in how your outfit looks.

The right **shape** complements your figure. Understanding your shape, accepting your shape, and starting to dress according to your body shape is key to looking your best. Whether you're skinny or full figured, learning what works best for your body type is important to create a balanced body. Clothing is either constructed along straight lines or along curved lines. The straight line gives a structured form, and curved lines give a more flexible shape.

Your Body Shape

If you have an **hourglass figure**, wearing soft lines will be to your advantage. Clothes that define your waistline and highlight your figure are best. It's important to stay away from clothes that hide your figure line. Whatever your body shape is your aim is to create a balanced-body look. For this body shape, straight skirts (pencil skirts) or an A-line cut with a definite waistband are good choices; so are fitted jackets with a waistline definition. Any style of dresses are good, but preferably those with a belt. Avoid boxy jackets, shapeless pants, baggy tops, and too many layers because they will make you look big and shapeless. Shapeless dresses, boxy jackets, baggy oversized sweaters, and too many layers of clothing will make you look fat.

If you have a **lean body type** with a small bust line, hips, and bottom, wearing layers is always a good choice. Jackets should be waisted with details to give you some volume. Skirts could be A-line or straight.

If you are **big chested**, start by getting a good fitting bra. The more structured your clothing is, the more proportionate your shape will become. The only way to get a longer, leaner line is to add volume to your bottom half. Jackets work well with some skin showing up by your face and a softly draped A-line skirt would balance the top half. A narrow skirt would emphasize the difference between your upper and lower halves. Also, wide leg pants could add the volume necessary to balance your upper part. Dresses need to have a waistline because if you are big chested, you lose your midsection and look heavier.

If you have a **big bottom**, it's important to focus your attention on your bottom half by choosing darker colors such as black, navy, brown or grey and more impactful colors on the top half to balance your body shape. Short jackets with a strong shoulder line that sit at the top of your hip would create a longer leg line and slim the hip. Also, jackets that are made of heavier fabrics would balance your overall look. A higher waist and slightly wide, straight-legged pants would create a longer leg line, which would give you a taller look. Dresses that have a soft A-line would balance your hip without adding too much volume.

A good rule to follow is to buy pieces that fit the largest area of your body comfortably and then tailor everything else to fit your slimmer body parts. A dress that is too tight around the hips or waist would not help flatter your figure, no matter how short you make the skirt. If the top portion of your body is big, balancing it with a bit more volume on the bottom half will give you that perfect balanced shape. Choosing wider or straight legged pants and an A-line skirt would help bring balance to your body. Remember, well constructed shapes generally enhance your figure, hide your imperfections, and hold you up in the right places. They make you look better than you look naked.

Colors can make you or break you. Your clothing needs to work in harmony and balance your natural coloring. The right color will complement and brighten your complexion. The colors that you wear closest to your face are the most important colors. They can either make you look younger and glowing, or they can make you look dreary. First, discover the colors that compliment your complexion.

If you have a **light complexion** (blond or ash brown hair), you can balance your coloring by wearing light to medium depth colors against your face and staying away from dark colors. If you like to wear black dresses, you have to make sure that you are going to use a scarf or jewelry around your neck to give you some color. Your make-up should complement your entire outfit as well. Aim for light and delicate.

If you have a **dark complexion** (black hair and eyes with dark toned skin), you can wear black, brown, or eggplant next to your face, but you need to balance it with lighter and brighter shades.

Never wear two light colors together, but you can wear two dark colors together.

If you have a **deep to warm complexion** and your hair has light brown tones, you can add camel, salmon, or terracotta to your dark colors to soften your look. The overall look of your make-up could be rich with a warm undertone.

If your coloring is a **warm brown with red-toned hair**, you need to balance it by choosing colors that have a warm yellow undertone. You will look good with colorings that are medium in depth, such as navy, grey, and brown. Warm them up with yellow, salmon, or peach.

If you have a **clear complexion with dark hair**, bright eyes, and skin that can be any tone from dark to light, you would look good in a contrast of light and dark colors. If you like to wear taupes, it's important to liven them up with brighter shades of yellow, light peach, light gold, coral, or clear salmon.

If you have **soft coloring** with dark blond hair and soft-colored eyes with no contrast between the color of your skin and hair, the best color clothing would be tone-on-tone with little contrast or tones of medium depth. Pale shades like soft whites or shell are your best colors.

Remember that dark colors make you look thinner. The preferred color in New York City, especially in the fall and winter, is black. Women cover themselves in black from top to toe. There are a few simple rules to wearing black. Leave some skin exposed around the neckline, and accessorize with jewelry. Having only dark colors in your closets limits your possibilities, and it could become dull. Add colors to your wardrobe, and don't be afraid to express yourself through your clothing.

Fabrics are important since different fabrics fall differently on your body. It's important to pay attention to the fabric's softness, flow, body, texture, and so on. Good textures to choose from are cotton, denim, silk, wool, crepe, and wool gabardine. These fabrics are wearable, comfortable, and they can enhance your shape. Stay away from fabrics that are too heavy on shine, texture, and composition, such as patent leather, sequins, tulles, and embroidery. They can make you look heavier then you are.

Present Dressing Style

Exercise III

How would you describe your overall look? Eclectic, organized, disorganized, neat, thoughtful, casual, elegant, simple, overmatched, relaxed, eye-catching, pretty, feminine, masculine, or other?

What type of shopper are you? Do you love shopping, dislike shopping, shop anxiously, shop thoughtlessly, bargain hunt, buy things that you like, buy only things that you need, shop creatively or thoughtfully, overshop or other?

How would you describe your work wardrobe? Conservative, eclectic, casual, sporty, formal, pretty, feminine, or other?

How would you describe your nonworking wardrobe? Elegant, matched, casual, coordinated, sporty, carefree, or other?

What types of accessories do you wear? Overmatched, casual, overdone, minimal, sporty, eclectic, creative, or other?

What types of shoes do you have? Casual, heels, flats, sandals, boots, or other?

What is your favorite color? What other colors do you wear?

Does your wardrobe reflect your present lifestyle? If your answer is yes, then keep on doing what you're doing because it works. But if the answer is no, then this is the time to adjust your clothing to fit more with who you are today.

At different points in our lives, we might feel differently about our looks and the clothing that we wear. Regardless of our age, if we enjoy looking good, we have acquired a taste for clothing, and we have discovered what does and what doesn't work for us. If, on the other hand, we had shown little interest in fashion, this is the time to start paying attention to our style and not get stuck in clothing that doesn't fit us or is uncomfortable, boring, outdated, and shapeless.

Clean Your Closet

"If your drawers and closets are overstuffed and messy, how can you expect the universe to deliver anything more? There is no space for more."

William Spear

"In order to become a smart shopper, clean your closet twice a year: spring and fall."

Lea Ausch

Open your closets and drawers, and examine every piece of clothing that you have. Try it all on, and decide which pieces you like and which ones you don't. Make two piles, one for yes and one for no. Don't hesitate to eliminate those pieces that you haven't worn in years or which still have the price tags attached to them. Keep all the clothes that you like, look good on you, and often wear. It feels good to recognize all the pieces that are hanging in your closet that look good on you.

Next, sort out the pieces that you like according to season, and put them back into your closets and drawers in an organized way that gives you easy access to your wardrobe. A clean and well organized closet helps you enjoy the clothes that you have.

Many times you might hear the saying, "Style cannot be learned." That's a myth because you continuously question what looks good on you. What makes you taller or slimmer? Which colors complement your complexion or eyes? What type of shoes should you wear, or what handbag or accessories should you use? The point that I am trying to make is that all these pieces that make up your style are learned. You learn by doing it. Practice makes you good at everything you do, including dressing.

Effortless Chic

What does it mean to dress effortlessly? It means to dress without trying too hard. Nothing ages us more than overmatched clothes. They look like we either try too hard or we don't try hard enough. Either way, it works against us. We need to forget about the old rules of dressing when everything was overmatched, when shoes and bags were the same color, when certain styles and colors we did not wear after a certain age, when whites were for summer and dark colors for winter, when we wore suits to our work place, when furs were worn only for the winter, when we did not mixed fabrics, colors or patterns.

All these old rules that governed our lives for thirty or forty years are very hard to change because they are familiar and we might not know anything else. But relinquishing our old habits and dressing more like we know what we are doing will make us look stylish and youthful again. We should look at dressing as an expression of our creativity, originality, and imagination. Remember, everything goes as long as it doesn't clash.

I can certainly relate to this rule of effortless dressing, since my clothes are a clear reflection of it. Every time I put an outfit together, I express my creativity and my passion for clothing. Adding a few new pieces to my wardrobe every season helps me evolve on my quest toward self-discovery. It allows me to look at myself with fresh new lenses and realize over and over again that I am only as old as I think and feel I am. Getting a more casual and unfinished look is my secret for looking stylish and youthful.

If we look around, we see that younger women dress more casually, simply, unassumingly and comfortably. Their outfits might be coordinated but not overmatched. Their style of dress is stylish, but also comfortable and sporty at the same time. So let's start by getting over our desire to overdress and overmatch by unleashing our creativity. We can replace suits with pants and tops. We can replace a formal dress with a more casual skirt and shirt. We can replace high heels with flats, especially if we are walking a lot. The only rule we need to follow is staying proportionate to our body shape. For example, long skirts will not look good on a petite woman. It will look overwhelming. A very tight fitted dress will not look good on a full-figured woman because it will accentuate her bulges. A very short skirt might not look good on someone who has fat legs.

Create Your Wardrobe

Basic pieces you should own are pants, skirts, jeans, dresses, jackets, tee shirts, shirts, cardigans, sweaters, suits, and accessories.

Jeans provide you with a youthful and sporty look. They are comfortable and easy to wear for either day or evening, depending on the look that you are trying to create. For example, a pair of jeans with a tee shirt is a sporty look for everyday wear, but with a dressier shirt it could be worn as an evening outfit. A good fitted pair of jeans with a dressy top has replaced the little black dress as a must-have staple. If you shy away from wearing jeans after a certain age, you deny yourself an important casual-sports look. The secret is finding the right fit, shape, and color since there are so many different brands to choose from.

The best fit are mid-low-rise boot cut jeans. The slight flare at the bottom is a good fit for most body types. The boot-cut jeans give you an optical illusion of longer legs, especially if you pair them with high heel shoes or boots. If you wear them with a high heel pump and a dressy top or a little fitted jacket, it's a classic look for almost every body type. It's a great look for the modern day women. The skinny jean gives you a straight and tight-looking silhouette. But unless you have a straight and skinny body, this style will look too tight on you. For a more formal look, you can wear a pair of trouser jeans, since they look like a pair of nice pants.

When it comes to colors, the most popular jeans are the true blue and the dark-washed jeans. Shoes and accessories make or break a pair of jeans. For example, straight legged jeans look the best with pumps or boots. The right length hits one quarter inch from the ground. The most important thing is making sure that it gives your butt a great shape. It's ideal to choose a smaller size pair of jeans, because jeans all tend to stretch and look baggy and shapeless. But you need enough room at the waistline to avoid the dreaded muffin top.

Pants are essential. Those that fit well are staples. They could be worn all year round and for all occasions. They are easy to wear and easily matched with anything you might have in your closets. A wool blend is nice for the winter months while a light color cotton is great for the summer months. For dressy pants the best rise is a midrise, which lies below your navel but above your hip.

There are many different options when it comes to pants such as wide leg, flare, straight, skinny, cropped, and baggy. You have to find the one that fits your body the best and gives you the best shape. Pants look good tailored but not tight. Length is important. Pants cannot be too long or not long enough, so it's advisable to try them on with shoes before you decide to hem them up.

Skirts are essential item in your wardrobe because, like pants, they are easy to wear and very versatile. There are many types of skirts and they all serve different functions. They could make you look more conservative, formal, and dressy, or they could create a sporty, carefree, and youthful look. Skirts come in different shapes, textures, length, colors, and fabrics. The most important rule is that they should fit comfortably at the waist. The best way to test a skirt is by sitting down. When you stand up, if the skirt remains bunched up around your hips, it's too small. When it comes to length, pencil or straight skirts should hit right below the knee. Knee length skirts should graze the top of your knee, and maxi skirts should stop just below the ground.

Once you have found the right length, you need to concentrate on the width of the skirt. Straight skirts are always a good choice. They make you look thinner and give your body a nice shape. If you want to go slimmer, a pencil skirt is your next choice. A little stretch in the fabric makes it easier to walk or sit in them. If you are afraid of looking fat in a straight skirt, the answer could be using a good tummy smoother. Remember, if your skirt is too tight, it makes you look heavier than you are, and it becomes a challenge to walk.

When it comes to shoes, the shorter your skirt, the lower your heel should be. It's all about the right proportion. If you choose a fuller and longer-looking skirt, a higher heel would give you a better proportion. Remember that size is not as important as the right fit and the right pair of shoes. The narrower the skirt, the sexier you will look. You can make a skirt short, but if it's too wide it's shapeless. The most popular skirt is the black pencil skirt. It's great with high heels, pumps, sandals, or boots.

Dresses are our preferred choice, and most of us have at least one dress hanging in our closets. No matter the day or the season, a dress that fits well will always make you look and feel fashionable. It's a good idea to have a black dress, which is perfect to wear in the summer with sandals or in the winter with high boots or booties.

Choosing the right style dress for your figure is important. If you choose a cut like an A-line flare, it will camouflage your hips and bottom well, but if you have a small waist, you need to show it off with a style that cuts in your midsection or to use a belt. If you have thick arms, a sleeveless dress would not be to your advantage, so you would need a dress with sleeves or a jacket. If you have a straight body shape, you would look good in a straight or fitted dress similar to the pencil skirt belted at the waist. Fit is key to making a dress look good on your body.

Dresses come in many different fabrics, from wool to cotton to silk to linen. Choosing the right fabric for your figure type is also important. For example, the heavier the fabric is, the heavier you will look. The lighter the fabric, the slimmer you will appear. Remember that the right fabric and fit can take off or add ten pounds to your look.

The best shoes for dresses are the sling back or classic pumps. The higher the heel, the better the dress looks. The heel has to be at least two inches high to give your legs a long appearance. Dresses could look good with flats or sandals if the dress is short enough to give you a balanced look. It's all about the right proportion. If you choose a fuller dress, a higher heel would give you the right balance.

Jackets and blazers are essential items to have in your wardrobe. Jackets could create a great outfit with either a skirt, pants, or a pair of jeans. The beauty of a blazer is that it can be used as formal or casual wear. A chic blazer could be unconstructed, fitted, oversized, or a classic fit.

The fit of blazers is important. The shoulder seam should sit at the outer edge of your shoulders. You need to make sure that the jacket is big enough so that you can move, stretch, and reach comfortably. If you are wearing a fitted jacket, it should not be too wide because then it might look boxy or heavy. If you want to wear it open, the blazer has to be tailored enough to maintain its shape.

There are essentially three basic styles that women wear: the classic fit blazer, the cropped blazer, and the boyfriend blazer. Classic blazers are good for formal occasions with a nice slim leg trouser or a pencil skirt. The cropped blazer helps balance out proportions of a flowing maxi dress and also looks fab with a high waist and belted skirt or a knee length dress. The boyfriend blazer is a more casual and cool look, which could be paired with a sequin top and a pair of jeans or a leather short skirt.

Suits are an essential addition to your wardrobe. The cool and modern way to wear a suit is to break it up. Wear the blazer with a different type of pants, skirt, jeans, or sleeveless dress, and wear the bottom with a shirt, sweater, or a simple tee or tank top. It's an easy way to create a modern suit for the modern-day woman. The double duty will be cost effective. If your job require you to wear a traditional suit, you could personalize it with jewelry and accessories. Suits also look good with a perfect stiletto. All these individual touches allow you to be creative and imaginative. As a result, the suit is not just a simple suit but rather your own creation.

Coats are a necessity for keeping warm but can also contribute to your style. A wool or cashmere-wool blend coat in black or any other rich color is a must for the fall, spring, and winter months. The best cut is the classic one or the straight one. Coats that need a belt usually are too bulky, and if you want to wear them open they become shapeless. The best length for a winter coat is either mid-thigh or to the knee. They look good with pants or over a dress. For the snowy season women prefer to wear water resistant quilted coats. The best choice is a sleeker version and not the very puffy down jackets that can make you heavier looking. A down style vest is another nice layer to have for the winter months.

Raincoats are usually worn in the rainy seasons of fall and spring. It's important to look for one that's light weight, water resistant, straight, and not belted if possible. The best length is to your knees. The best colors to choose from are black, taupe, olive, or light brown because they are easy to wear with almost everything.

Shirts and tops must fit well and not to be too tight on your chest or back. You don't want any bulges on your back. The back should lie smooth without showing any bumps or that you're wearing slimming undergarments. A poorly fitting bra can led to unattractive bulges under any shirt.

The most common and versatile tops are tee shirts. They come with long sleeves, short sleeves, or no sleeves. They are great by themselves or layered over a tank top. Tee shirts are made from many different fabrics, such as cotton, silk, or some kind of blend. Tee shirts work well under blazers, cardigans, or just by themselves.

In the winter and cool summer nights a comfortable layer is just the right thing to have. Cardigans do nicely. There is something special about being covered by a cashmere, wool, or wool-blend sweater. Sweaters are a good option to wear over almost anything including a sleeveless dress. A sweater is good with pants and skirts and can be worn all year around.

By now you should feel that you have acquired a basic grasp on what you need to build a balanced and accommodating wardrobe. Don't feel pressure to go out and fill any gaps you identified all at once. Part of the fun in building a personal wardrobe is finding the perfect pieces over time. Jot down any items that are missing from your wardrobe. Keep the list in mind as you shop or browse online, and fill in your missing pieces as you find them. Don't put any pressure on yourself.

Body Shapewear

Beneath your great jeans or a jersey dress lies a good body shaper. Body shapers lift, smooth, mold, and shape, and they can easily hide ten pounds. Once you get to your middle age your demand for good underwear increases. As you age, even the thinnest among us gets back fat and muffin tops. When you look good in an outfit, it's not its size that counts but rather its shape. If an outfit looks good on you, it means that it fits you well, and it facilitates your body shape. It accentuates your good features and camouflages your less perfect areas. So familiarizing yourself with your body shape is important.

Bras can make your outfit look great or ruin it. When you are trying on bras, it's important to get the full picture of how they will look underneath your outfit. Putting on a top over the bra will help you judge if the bra gives you the shape that you would like.

There are many different styles and sizes of bras. There are three important areas that you need to consider when shopping for a bra: cup size, straps and support. You need to determine if your bra is hoisting you high enough; otherwise it will not create a good fit for your tops. A bra that fits can make you look thinner, creating a longer and leaner torso. The cup size should be roomy for your entire breast. The right size cup should lay flat on your entire breast without extra material, and your breast should not hang over the cup. The back of your bra should sit in the middle of your back.

Panties cannot be too lose or too tight. Finding the right fit, especially under straight skirts and fitted pants, is important. Eliminate visible panty lines by ensuring that the elastic doesn't cut into your flesh. Panties that are the closest color to your skin will blend in with your skin. If you need tummy control, it's important to make sure that they fit well and that your flesh doesn't roll over the top when you sit down. If you have a lot of belly fat, shapewear instead of regular underwear could help you minimize your belly rolls.

Problem Areas

Arm flab can be hard to hide if you fall in love with a little black sleeveless dress. But you can easily throw over it a short fitted jacket, cardigan, wrap, or shawl. Flabby arms do not mean that you are overweight. They mean that you need to work on your triceps. Weight-bearing exercises, such as picking up dumbbells or grocery bags a few times a week, would strengthen your muscle mass, increase your metabolism, and improve your posture.

Back fat, tummy overhang, or bra rolls are common among middle-aged women. Back fat can be eliminated by wearing a fitting bra that eradicates those bulges. For your muffin tops or for your dress-thinner strategy, you can wear a high-waist body shaper. You should stay away from tops that are tight or fit snug on your bust. Belly fat can be helped by using good tummy control underwear. It's important to stay away from dresses without a waistline because they don't give you a break at the center to attract your eyes, and you will look shapeless. A belt or a wasted dress will immediately give your shape a sleeker line through your middle. Using layering to hide your bulges does not work because it adds pounds across your middle.

Big booties are easy to deal with using good shapewear. Choosing the right type of clothes that are loose enough to easily flow over your entire back side can solve your problem. Use jackets, cardigans, and tunics that can cover your butt. Make sure that they are not too heavy because they could add volume to your butt. Keep your back simple and subdued so as not to attract more attention to your butt.

Accessories

Shoes

By far accessories are the easiest way to spruce up your outfits and update your wardrobe. Most women love shoes and handbags. They are the hallmark of our wardrobe. What has fueled this fire for more and more shoes is that shoe manufacturers offer new styles and must-have shoes every season. No doubt, there is a large discrepancy between how many pairs of shoes you own and how many you actually wear. If you look through your shoe racks, you are bound to find many pairs of shoes that you have not worn in years.

Shoes have to be comfortable; otherwise you walk funny. Before buying a pair of shoes you have to pay attention to your clothes to be able to determine what kind of shoes would go best with your outfits. Shoes can make an outfit look great, or they can ruin it. The most popular types of shoes are pumps, high heels, platforms, Mary Jane fitted knee-high boots, ankle boots, sneakers, and walking shoes. The thicker the heel, the easier is for you to walk in them.

When you are shopping for shoes, the fit is the number one concern. It's a good idea to get your feet measured to assess your size. You also need to test the fit by standing up and walking with them for a few minutes in the store to make sure that they fit properly. When it comes to the height of the heels, you need to walk for a few minutes to see if you feel comfortable enough in the height. The safest height is two to three inches. Anything higher might throw you off balance, throwing your body weight forward and exerting a lot of pressure on the ball of your feet. You need to find the right heel and still look stylish without going to high.

Shoes give your outfits a little punk look. When wearing them with pants, it's important to keep the color the same so it will give you a longer look. For example, a pair of black skinny pants tucked into a black boot will elongate your legs and make you feel fabulous at the same time. When wearing shoes with skirts, you should use black opaque tights to keep the line going. Knee boots look good with skirts or dresses. As your skirts gets shorter, your boots get higher.

Sandals or wedges are ideal for the summer months. They come in many different styles and materials. Again, you need to choose the one that goes well with your outfit. Sandals must fit you perfectly. No part of your foot should spill over the side, the back, or the front. You also need to make sure that your feet are pedicured.

Another important component of your leg wear is tights. If you are wearing a short skirt or dress, showing leg is a youthful look. Wearing no pantyhose is the best look. But if you feel uncomfortable with showing so much leg, you can put on an ultra-sheer, flesh-colored pantyhose. Solid tights are a choice for winter and fall months. Remember, it's important that the shades of your pantyhose should easily blend with your skirts and shoes to create the illusion of longer legs. Control top pantyhose serve as a good control and create a smoother line under your clothes. For example, black tights go well with black boots or a black pump, so our eyes see one sleek leg line.

Handbags can make you look great or can ruin your look. A good handbag is an indicator of your personal style. Handbags come in different styles and sizes. It's important to get a bag that is appropriate for your body type, one that looks good on you and serves your needs. There is nothing worse than carrying a very large handbag crammed full of stuff.

Your bag should not drag you down or look too overwhelming. Consider what you actually use on a daily basis from your bag. Keep it minimal, like a wallet, phone, keys, a pen, some make-up, a daily planner, and maybe a snack. It's important to stay away from the bag-lady look. It's not attractive to carry a big, bulky bag with your whole life inside, especially as you age. It pulls you down, and it gives you neck, back and shoulder problems.

Jewelry and Belts

The key objective is to keep a balance between your jewelry and clothing. If your jewelry is bulky, you need to keep your clothing simple. If you are wearing a statement, piece you need to keep your focus on that piece. Adding more would deflect attention from your main piece. If you are wearing simple, delicate jewelry, you can wear more than one piece. But the days of buying a matching necklace, earring, and bracelet set are over. Mixing up your jewelry will give you a fresher, younger look. When used properly, each piece of jewelry can enhance your outfit and add more zest to it. Whether it's a scarf, belt, hair tie, or headband, it can add more creativity to your outfit. The simple rule, less is more, applies to your accessories as well.

Glasses

Adding the right pair of glasses will communicate your personal style more strongly than anything else because glasses cover a big part of your face. Frames are strong fashion statements. Boring frames, metal rims, half-glasses, or hanging chains make us look older, stale, and outdated. It's important to stay away from rimless glasses. They look too grandmotherly. Thin metal frames are too boring, and round frames are too old and collegiate looking.

Because of their importance on your face, eyeglasses can have a powerful impact on your looks. They are visible every waking hour of your day. It's important to update your glasses once a year when you get your vision checked. It will refresh your look.

Most of us look good in a frame that is horizontal with a small upward tilt at the outer edges. Any downturned frame will make your face look sad and droopy. Frames come in different colors. Warm colors bring softness to your face, while metal frames give you a cold look. Frame colors should blend in well with your hair and eye color. The magic is to find a frame that brings brightness to your face.

Your outside appearance, including your make-up, hair, clothing, and accessories is a wonderful tool that you can manipulate to present yourself to your advantage regardless of your age, size, shape, or height by simply recognizing your physical assets and limitations. You need to explore the best ways in which your outer look can be used to draw attention to your assets and camouflage your imperfections. If you take some time and effort, you can alter at least one area of your looks, and slowly other areas will follow. You are worth taking care of yourself.

Achieving a youthful look might not be as hard as you might think at your age. It takes some courage, creativity, and guidance, which I hope this chapter provides. You need to look at yourself with a new pair of lenses that allow you to see clearly those things you can change and those you cannot. It's time to let go, unleash your creativity, and free yourself from the prison that you blindly created for yourself. Soon you will feel more comfortable with yourself because it will reflect your true self today.

CHAPTER IX

Simplify and Rightsize Your Life

> "When you eliminate the impossible, whatever remains—however improbable—must be the truth".
>
> Sir Arthur Doyle (1859-1930)

> "All true things must change, and only that which changes remains true".
>
> Carl Jung

This book is built on the premise that change is a prerequisite for a healthy life, and since we all possess the inner power to bring it about, we can overcome the adversities that might come our way. We have the power over our health by eating well and exercising. We can improve the power of our brain by using it. We can improve our level of income by getting an education. We can increase our education level by going back to school or by consciously attending the school of life. We can improve our self-confidence by learning how to trust our abilities. We can improve our outer appearance by paying attention to our self-grooming. It's time to examine other areas of our lives that might need changes.

Change, anim-morphosis, at any age is important for both our mental and physical health. Middle age is a perfect time to reflect upon our lives, celebrate the things that work well, and change those that no longer work. Many times we are too scared—locked into our old habits, unable to move on with our lives—and we make up reasons or excuses for why we cannot change. We become stuck, and our aging process accelerates at a much faster rate.

Many of our habits are difficult to break because they have been hard wired by our society. For example, we have been encouraged throughout our lives to be productive. We have adopted this message and now it is habit. But when the very habits that our society rewards us for, like productivity, begin depleting our resources, it makes for a tough environment to change. We all know that stress is bad for our health, but the overwork that causes stress seems to be a socially desirable thing, so we adopt it without questioning. In fact, overwork is a toxic addiction that can make us both physically and mentally burned out, stressed, anxious, and prone to disease.

This chapter raises the possibility that some areas of our lives might need simplifying. Simplifying your life and carrying a lighter load will set you free from the burdens that you might be carrying on your shoulders. Think of life as a suitcase: the more you pack, the heavier it becomes and the harder it is to carry. This chapter's focus is learning to recognize this reality and change the way we travel through life. Now, ask yourself: How do I pack the suitcase called my life?

Previous chapters dealt is our physical and mental fitness as a prerequisite for keeping us vigorous and functioning, our nutrition and its many benefits for our physical and mental health, and our renewed sense of self and appearance. This chapter continues to expand our horizons in other areas of our lives that might need some changes. This is our chance to develop a perfect fit between what we have and what we could have. With a little effort and planning we can achieve the life that we have envisioned for ourselves.

Rightsizing our lives is a conscious, practical, and psychological evaluation of the way we live. This re-evaluation can come at any point in our lives. It could be triggered by getting bored with our job, being stuck in a bad relationship, or by reading this book that opens our minds to new possibilities. We need to put on a fresh pair of lenses through which we can see clearly how we want to live the rest of our lives. This conscious process helps us carve out new visions and realities.

Our lives do not just happen. They're designed by us. We are the ones that create our successes and failures, our sadness and happiness, our fears and courage, our worries and concerns, our stress and calm, our actions and inactions. Now it's time to redirect our attention and rewrite our life script any way and any time we desire. Our level of self-awareness, acceptance, motivation, and confidence in our abilities will dictate the direction in which we will proceed.

Each day we are faced with challenges, opportunities, and conflicts that need to be dealt with. We can either be proactive and focus our efforts on solutions, or we can be reactive and stuck. For example, by focusing our efforts on things that are out of our control, we are wasting our energy on wishful thinking, excuses, long explanations, blame, and inaction. We need to take responsibility for our life and move toward promoting our well-being.

All changes begin with our acknowledgement that the power of transformation comes from within us. We have the power to change the things that don't work well in our lives and to stop discouraging ourselves from taking any personal responsibility.

My moment of renewal and re-discovery came soon after I lost my first husband some twenty-five years ago to cancer. I felt a strong sense of panic and anxiety about my life and my existence. I felt stuck. My needs, visions, and aspirations for the future were not met, and I needed something different. But what was it? Overwhelming questions cluttered my mind. Where would I live? With whom would I live? Would I reopen my practice or continue my job as a university professor? How would I deal with my finances? Would I remarry some day? All these questions overwhelmed me, but at the same time they excited me, and I knew that they needed my attention.

I felt disconnected and out of balance both internally as well as socially. Throughout my marriage, I became what my husband wanted me to be and adopted his lifestyle, values, and strong religious beliefs. Now it was my time to find out who I was underneath the roles of daughter, wife, mother, and grandmother. I needed to find my own way in life.

As my belief in myself grew stronger, I was able to move toward new discoveries and new, exciting experiences. A whole world opened up, which led me to a complete anim-morphosis in many areas of my life. As I started making changes, my life became simpler, easier, and more enjoyable. I got rid of a lot of garbage that cluttered my life for many years, including bad relationships, family, work, finances, and my inner turmoil. All this clutter distracted and kept me stuck for many years.

Cleaning the toxicity out of my life involved cleaning my gut, my brain, my nutrition, my environment, and my body. Slowly, I was able to find some of the obstacles that stood in my way and remove them one by one. It was quite a demanding job and at times stressful, but soon I realized that taking action, good or bad, was better than staying stuck in my own misery. It was scary to walk on this new, unfamiliar path, but trust me it was worth the trip.

Your Clutter

Exercise I

Get in touch with your clutter.

Do you see clutter in your life? Is there chaos, stress or toxicity?

Where do you see clutter?

Does it hinder your life? How?

Are you ready to do something about it?

Clutter in any area of your life makes your life harder. You are carrying a heavier load filled with both internal and external turmoil, chaos, stress, disorder, toxic relationships, job dissatisfaction, and a constant feeling of anxiety. All this turmoil holds you back from enjoying your life. The lighter your life's load, the clearer your mind will be and the easier all your decision making will become.

You need to de-clutter both your inner and outer life. Get rid of self-sabotaging behavior, judgments, criticisms, self-pity, insecurities, fears, worries, stress, self-doubts, regrets, and guilt. Eliminate your outer clutter, including negative work experiences, bad relationships, financial chaos, over-commitment, and a chaotic home environment. Clutter on the outside is often a reflection of clutter on your inside. This strong interconnection between your inner and outer life serves as a glue to your existence.

The hardest job most of us face is having an honest self-evaluation, which begins by breaking out of our habitual patterns of thinking and acting. Our past experiences form the basic foundation of our habits. Those old habits might lock us into inaction, control, rigidity, fear, worry, stress, insecurity, and self-doubt. All these are major impediments to our growth. We need to become aware of the root causes of our behaviors so we can start rightsizing our inner and outer lives and restore balance.

Your Habitual Thinking

We have all heard the saying "humans are creatures of habit." This means that we often conduct our lives on autopilot. This would explain why some of us are stuck while others are not, why some of us suffer one personal rejection after another while others do not, why some of us are locked in a dead-end job while others are not. Most of us suspect an assortment of reasons for our unhappy existence, but rarely do we suspect the culprit to be nothing more than our bad habits. We feel victimized by life, looking to be saved from our own despair and self-inflicted misery.

But let's be honest: most of us are not looking for change. We want to become better neurotics, better at managing our lives. For example, the workaholic is not looking to slow down, just to get a few good nights of sleep. The perfectionist wants to become more perfect without the anxiety that being perfect creates. How many time have you said to yourself, "I really have to change," only to continue on the same path. One part of our struggle is caused by our incessant rituals. Over time we get attached to them, including our problems, conflicts, stress, worry, insecurity and control. As difficult as our life is, we hold on to them because they are familiar and feel safe to us.

The simple fact that we are not born unhappy, insecure, stressed, angry, or frustrated seems to escape our awareness. Our lives, whether easy or difficult, are our own creation that originated from our past experiences. It's the result of our learned patterns of perception. If all our problems are learned, then the good news is that we can unlearn them as well. It's time to stop being unhappy, stressed, anxious, angry, or miserable and start learning how to jump-start our lives. We can create the life we want for ourselves because this power is within us. We just need to learn how to access it and use it.

No matter how destructive our habits are, they cannot hurt us if we stop feeding them. How do we feed our habits? Every time we doubt ourselves or feel anxious or stressed, we are throwing our habits crumbs of our insecurity and thereby strengthening them. We have to give up our habituated patterns of thinking and start healing ourselves. This is about being proactive, taking charge of our lives by empowering ourselves to take control of our behaviors. We need to cultivate our inborn capacity for happiness. By nature, we are creative, flexible, and easily adaptable, and we were that way in our childhood years. We just need to reconnect with that side of our being and recapture the energy and enthusiasm of our youth.

In my case, only after I learned to overcome my impediments in life, including, anger, stress, frustration, fear, insecurity, and toxic relationships, was I able to move from a very controlled thinking to a more spontaneous understanding of what I needed in my life. I learned to let go of my idea of how things should be. I started to understand that my reality is derived from my own thought system, and since we are all creating our own realities via our individual thought systems, our lives become a true reflection of those realities.

I understood the principle of separate realities. Once I became aware of the powerful connection between my thinking and my experiences, as well as that of others, I was able to let go of many of my negative habitual thinking patterns and become more accepting and understanding of myself and others.

Our thought system contains all the information we have accumulated over our lifetime. It's this past information that our thought system uses to interpret the significance of everything that happens in our lives. This means that our thought system is the source of our conditioned thoughts. When we rely on conditioned thoughts, we are thinking in a habitual manner and relying on our usual way of seeing things. Our thoughts contain our own view of the way life is, which leads us to believe that we are realistic and the way we see life is really the way it is.

With this basic understanding, we can begin to see and sense the value in others' points of view. What we used to interpret as criticism, we now understand as nothing more than an opinion from another person's point of view, which originated from their own thought system. As a result, we can eliminate being angry or frustrated at others who don't see things our way and accept conflict as originating from a different system of thoughts.

Our belief system has been with us all our lives. It was created in the past where it might have served us well, but now it could be moving us in the wrong direction. We need to start listening to the things we say to ourselves today and stay away from thoughts and beliefs that caused us pain and problems in the past. For example, if we know that we have an allergy to peanuts, we will stay away from them. The same principle applies to our thoughts. If we know that certain thoughts cause us pain, we need to stay away from them. Our thoughts become our resistance to change. We might use different excuses to hold on to them and explain our inaction. We may think, "I am too old," "There is nothing wrong with my life," "Everyone around me has problems," or "What good would it be to change at my age?"

If our life is unpleasant, we are creating our own misery via our thought system. Once we stop focusing on our problems, we will start experiencing a healthier perspective on life. Albert Einstein once said, "The solution to a problem will never come about from the same level of understanding that created the problem in the first place. " This means that we need to step back from our problem in order to find the solution. Just stop thinking about it.

The more we focus on our negative thoughts, the more real they will seem to be. Staying positive; avoiding negativity (like complaining, worrying, comparing, criticizing); getting in touch with our sense of adventure, excitement, and creativity; being proactive and taking responsibility for our own lives without blame, excuses, or procrastination: these will be our strongest allies toward change, new learning, and renewal.

A simple formula for change is as follows:

Positive Thinking + Varying Degrees of Emotions = All the Things We Have Attracted

This formula means that what we have focused on and how we use it is what we have got. If our attention is focused on things that need to be fixed, meaning things we don't want, we produce negative tension in our lives. So whatever we have right now is simply the result of how we distributed our energy in days gone by, accepting it as reality. When we focus our attention on "don't wants," it means we are holding on to them by our very thoughts. The only way to stop the messes in our lives is by not focusing on them, letting go of our preoccupation with "what we don't want," and changing those things to "wants."

It's time to get to work and get real with ourselves. No more cons, lies, or masks. We need to discover our real self that has been hiding behind the walls that we have built to defend ourselves from pain, discomfort, stress, shame, guilt, and so on. It's time for truth and clarity about ourselves and our lives. This honesty will give us access to power we never thought possible. Getting real with ourselves lies at the foundation of our existence. To have a different life, we need to be different, do different, and think different. Our commitment to act differently will help us get the life that we want, since by now we know that our old actions will only give us the same old results.

The Power of Reinventing Yourself

As children we learn about ourselves by the reactions of our parents, teachers, family, and community. These early experiences have a big impact, and their effects are felt throughout our lives. If we grow up in an overly critical environment, then we internalize many negative views about ourselves and those around us. But if we had the good fortune to grow up in a supportive and accepting environment, our lives will reflect that reality. Most of the time as adults we still treat ourselves the way our parents did.

Let's remember that our parents taught us what they learned from their own parents. For example, if your mother did not respect herself, it would have been impossible for her to teach you how to respect yourself. We formed our beliefs as young children and then we moved through life creating experiences to match those beliefs. We recreated those experiences again and again, and soon they became our habits.

However, that was the past, and now we need to move forward toward the future. The only important thing right now is what we think today, since those are the thoughts that create our future. Our past is over. Just think how crazy it is for us to punish ourselves today because someone hurt us in the past. We need to start a healthy relationship with ourselves and create a nurturing environment that we might not have experienced growing up in our family.

Taking care of ourselves is the basis for our physical and mental health. We cannot nurture others if we don't take care of our needs first. When we nurture others from a place of fullness, they feel renewed, and we don't feel depleted or used since we have a lot to give. Self-nurturing, taking care of ourselves, is not self-indulgent but rather essential for our survival.

In many societies, women we have been discouraged from taking care of their needs and encouraged to take care of others. We either ended up believing that we don't deserve self-care, or we take care of ourselves and feel guilty about it. We need to change these distortions that we have internalized and accepted as reality and to replace them with new realities and new experiences.

We value the importance of our contribution to our family and social group, but we cannot put it above the value of ourselves. It's hard to shed the automatic caretaking roles that have won us much praise throughout the years, let alone replace them with new beliefs and behaviors associated with taking our lives as seriously as we take those of others.

Nurturing ourselves means empowerment and self-acceptance. We can accept the fact that we no longer demand sustenance and happiness from others, because we can give it to ourselves. This freedom to choose and to be in charge of our lives feels extremely nurturing. To stay on the right track, we need to ask ourselves from time to time what we need for ourselves.

Both self-acceptance and self-compassion are the key elements we need for any positive changes to occur in our lives. If we master self-acceptance, we will stop ourselves from being overly critical, and all the negativity that created our self-doubt, stress, worry, fear, and anxiety, locking us into the very pattern we are trying to change, will be gone from our lives. Once we learn to accept ourselves we will be able to accept others around us and improve our relationships.

Eliminate Your Inner Toxicities

By eliminating our inner toxicities we free ourselves from some of the major impediments that stagnated our growth, such as control, fear, shame, pain, guilt, and stress. At the same time, we open ways to new discoveries by cultivating flexibility, resilience, and confidence.

All changes come hard. We need to be vigilant about our old habitual thinking and disarm those thoughts as they occurs. The good news is that your current thoughts are totally under your control. The past is over and cannot be changed, but the present is right here and it's totally within your control. Stop dwelling on what you don't want because you create more of it. You must realize that the same patterns of thinking that get you where you are today will not get you where you want to go. You need to defend yourself against all types of inner toxicities since they are all insecurity- and control-driven as well as resistant to change.

Your Impediments

Control is one of our major impediment driven by our insecurities, fears, worries, self-doubt, hostilities, and anger. All these are insecurity-driven attempts to control our lives. When we lose control, we try to get more of it by using our insecurities, which gives us an artificial false sense of security. We embrace insecurity by thinking that control is the glue that keeps our lives from crumbling. If insecurity is at the root of our problems, then trying to control our lives is the weed that grows from it and sooner or later will overrun our lives with worry, fear, and self-doubt.

Many times we buy into the myth that society sells us, which says that aging is associated with rigidity and control while youth is associated with flexibility and creativity. If we buy into this myth, then we lock ourselves in with our old habitual thinking, and there is no room for change. Both flexibility and creativity are learned behaviors. We can learn them at any age. By cultivating our flexibility with awareness, we can renew ourselves and slow down our aging process. Infinite flexibility and creativity is our antidote and nutrition for longevity and health.

The essence of flexibility is learning to let go of things that hinder our lives, whether they are nutrition, lack of activity, lack of sleep, bad relationships, or a dead end job. We can start relinquishing and let our lives evolve. Attempting to stop change by holding on is fighting the natural forces of evolution. The wear and tear born of our resistance accelerates our aging process and robs us of our health. We need to start trusting ourselves, which means creating a willingness to believe in ourselves and take risks.

Fear. To some degree we are all afraid of change since we cannot predict the future and change implies uncertainty. For example, the fear of ending a bad relationship and the uncertainty it creates may make us believe being alone is worse. We might question our ability to be alone or to meet someone else. Our brain likes predictability and control. When things are uncertain, our brain attempts to make up an ending with its own narrative. The problem is that most of the time the ending is negative, and this negativity leads to problems reinforcing our fear to the point that we become paralyzed.

Fear is a self-destructive emotion that deals a fatal blow to our confidence. If we are afraid, it's impossible to have the positive mental attitude essential for successful living. By giving into our thoughts of failure, we are impelled to fail. Only positive mental attitudes can help us overcome our fears by reinforcing our beliefs until we consciously accept them as facts.

Worry is another strong impediment, a habit of anticipated chaos, problems, conflicts, and danger causing us stress and misery. We all worry sometimes, so we might think that is part of our nature. But it's not, and it's not real. Worry in anticipation of something that has not happened but that might go wrong is irrational thinking that torments us. "What if thinking" deals with fiction and not reality. Worry is a form of control over things that have not happened and are out of our control. How many times have we told someone, or someone has told us, to stop making mountains out of molehills? Unfortunately, if worry has become our reflex mountain-making, then it's what we do best and we will continue doing it.

Replacing worry, which is compulsive and self-destructive, with concern, which is reality-based, will help us move toward motivation and courage. Concern deals with reality, and it's an honest assessment of actual problems. We can replace fear and worry, which lead to inaction, with courage and confidence, which promote action and change.

Shame, regrets, and guilt are other impediments that hinder our growth. Both shame and guilt were internalized early in our childhood years when a significant adult shamed us with insults, negativity, criticism, and discouragement. If we grew up in a family where there was a lot of criticism or negativity, we internalized it, and we tend to recreate it in our adult lives, creating a self-defeating life for ourselves. We punish ourselves the same way as our parents did. We begin to believe we aren't good enough, and we tell ourselves that repeatedly.

Shame and guilt are those dangerous feelings that make us feel small, flawed, invisible, and just not good enough. Both shame and guilt are our fear of not being accepted and loved. They make us feel unworthy. If anyone will hear our story, they will think less of us, won't accept us or like us. When something shaming happens to us it further reinforces our feeling, keeping us locked up. The good news is that shame loses some of its power when it's spoken. So talking about it with people we trust relieves our shame. Owning our own stories is the best shame-resistance technique that we have.

When we don't deal with our shame, we either move away from people, hide, keep secrets, or take the opposite approach by trying to gain more power over others by being aggressive or using shame tactics. The easiest way to address our feelings of shame is by cultivating awareness and recognizing our symptoms as they occur, such as fast heart rates, becoming red in the face, and getting dry mouth or sweaty palms.

Guilt is just as powerful and toxic as shame, but its effects can be positive at times. Shame, however, always destroys us. When we apologize for our behavior and we replace our negative behavior with a positive one, our guilt is our motivator, not shame. Shame destroys that part of us that thinks we can change or do things differently. Many times shame will lead us to self-destructive behaviors. For example, when we use shame self-talk such as "I am bad," it's much more destructive than guilt self-talk, such as "I did something bad." Shame tells us that we are inherently worthless and unlovable.

Shame's first cousin is **perfectionism**. Wherever perfectionism exists, shame is present as well. Perfectionism is not the same thing as striving to be our best. It's not about self-improvement; it's about trying to earn approval and acceptance. "If I look perfect, I can avoid being judged." But this kind of thought is self-destructive because perfectionism is an unattainable goal, and we just set ourselves up to fail: "It's my fault. I am not good enough." However seductive the notion of being perfect may be, it's nothing more than a lifelong prison to control self-loathing. For the perfectionist, a very thin line separates happiness from pain and chaos.

Regrets. Most of the time we don't realize the powerful effects that regrets have on us. Some regrets for roads not explored, goals not accomplished, or opportunities missed are normal, but too many regrets can feel painful, especially in middle age, when we might ask ourselves if our goals are still viable.

To attack our regrets, we must change our thinking about upsetting situations to more favorable outcomes. In his landmark book, *A Guide to Rational Living and Feeling Better* (1960), Albert Ellis argued that changing our thinking about upsetting situations more favorably can lead us to more productive behavior. Attacking our fears by thinking differently about our lives can help us move forward and turn our inactions into positive life-enhancing actions.

To fight our inner toxicities that cause distortions and unhappiness in our lives, we need to become aware of our vulnerabilities, practice self-acceptance, self-compassion, resilience, and strengthen our confidence in our abilities. Resilience is our ability to overcome adversities.

Resilient people are more positive, stronger, believe that things will get better, find things to be happy about, don't give up, have a sense of purpose, and believe that they can make a difference. Ultimately, resilience is a mind-set of seeing ourselves victorious and as survivors rather than a victims. It's the exact opposite of feeling shame, where we see our flawed selves.

Most of us engage in behaviors that we find safe to guard ourselves against vulnerability. But many times these behaviors are fueled by our misguided beliefs, which stop the flow of positive thinking, feeling, and action. When we deny ourselves the darker side of life, we also deny ourselves the lighter side, sabotaging our resilience, courage, and confidence.

Both courage and confidence are our strongest allies for overcoming our impediments. They're developed when we start trusting our abilities to bring about positive changes in our lives. We all know that to succeed at anything we must stay on task and fight our demons. To change our self-sabotaging behavior, we have to get off autopilot and stop doing the same things over and over again.

We need to reach outside our comfort zone and rock the boat. Once we decide on our course of action, our sailing becomes easier and everything is well within our reach.

Confidence in our ability to change those things that no longer work in our lives will keep us on the right track. It will strengthen our resolve to fight off all negativity with positive affirmations. Our negative voice tries to discourage us from making any changes and venturing into unfamiliar territories. It keeps us complacent and stuck. When our lives become overwhelming, it's really easy to shut down, not take a hard look around us, and be unaccountable for our thinking, acting and feeling.

In dealing with our inner toxicities, we need to familiarize ourselves with one of our worst enemies: stress. Stress is not something that just happens to us; rather, it is something that we create from within with our thoughts and perceptions. We decide what is going to be stressful. But in reality the more we try to think about our stresses or attempt to change them, the worse they will become because we believe that stress exists outside of ourselves.

If we don't understand where our stress originates, we look for ways to change the source. Let's take our job as an example. If we cannot change our circumstances, in this instance our job, than we continue to use it as our excuse for being stressed and unhappy. All this leads us to more stress and unhappiness. But it's not our job or the busy schedule that created our stress. Rather, it's our perception of the situation, and our thoughts about our job, that stressed us out.

If our stress is created by our thoughts, to get rid of our stress we need to understand that it's our perception of the situation that causes our stress. So it's not the busy schedules that we have, but rather the thinking about the schedule that stresses us out. Once we understand that there is no such thing as stress, only stressful thinking, we can start taking responsibility of our own lives and maintain more calm, even when things get hard.

Let's learn not to blow things up in our minds. Healthy psychological functioning does not allow us to clutter our minds with anger, stress, or frustration; instead, it allows us to see with a clear head the best solution possible given the facts. Unhealthy psychological functioning can turn even the smallest event into a stressful situation.

Let's not minimize our problems; they are real. But once we master a sense of inner peace, our problems won't stop us from enjoying our lives. When we learn to live with less stress, less overthinking, and in a more peaceful state of mind, our quality of life will improve and we can actually think better, easier, clearer and faster.

Eliminate Your Outer Clutter

Now that we have familiarized ourselves with some of our inner clutter, it's time to examine our outer clutter that might cause us unhappiness and hinder our dreams. Too often we get distracted by our daily routines or by drama and we lose our focus, failing to engage in the most important parts of our lives. We clutter our lives with stuff, such as being too busy, overcommitted, overworked, or surrounded with toxic relationships keeping us from things that truly matter. We lose the sense of certainty that creates our winner's edge, resulting in many conflicts and agendas being pushed aside and not dealt with. We end up living in a way that is out of sync with who we really are, causing us missed opportunities and regrets.

As we get into our middle-age years, we start regretting our missed opportunities without realizing that we can still accomplish them with the inner power that lies dormant within us. We just need to de-clutter our lives to find this power, access it, and unleash it. At this point in our lives we need to ask ourselves, what would our lives be like if we focus more on ourselves and on the people that are important to us? We have arrived at an important cross roads in our lives, middle age, where wasting our lives with people and situations that serve us negativity is just plain stupid.

Toxicity in any area of our lives distracts and derails us from staying focused to achieve our goals. Too many distractions, too much chaos, can overwhelm us and derail us. Too much negativity caused by toxic people and situations could cause us stress, anxiety, self-doubt, and inaction as well as health problems. This is the time to do something about it.

Toxic people create toxic environments. Just as our own negativity can make us sick, so does the negativity that we experience from our outside environment. As George Orwell so eloquently put it, "The great enemy of clear language is insincerity." Researchers have found that toxic people, people with critical, insincere, phony social behavior, have a damaging effect on our health and could cause eating disorders, insomnia, low self-esteem, stress, anger, depression, and a generalized state of anxiety.

When we are locked in difficult relationships or we are surrounded by friends who are critical and discouraging of us, our energy gets depleted and we become stressed, anxious, and miserable. On the other hand, there is no mystery to the fact that positive relationships make us feel better and more optimistic about ourselves. People who are positive in our lives are encouraging of our dreams, listen well, make positive, encouraging, and useful comments and are eager to hear good news in our lives.

We have all heard the expression, "With friends like these, who needs enemies." There is nothing so disheartening as when someone who we trust betrays us. Sometimes we tolerate people and call them friends when they are anything but. Perhaps we feel sorry for them because their lives didn't turn out as well as ours, or we grew up with them. No matter how we rationalize it, these people cause us grief, pain, and severe disappointment by disrespecting us and betraying our trust.

A friend is someone who will never break a confidence and will defend us. Friends do not try to compete with us, but rather they are generous, sensitive, and accepting. A true friend openly and honestly shares thoughts and feelings and does not judge. Anyone who has less than these characteristics is not a true friend.

Toxic People

Exercise II

This exercise will focus your attention on all the toxic people that you have surrounded yourself with.

1. Are there toxic people in your life? Who are they?
2. Do you feel emotionally drained after spending time with them?
3. Do you feel like running away from them?
4. Are you in a bad mood, stressed, or unhappy after spending time with them?
5. Are they being judgmental, argumentative, sarcastic, dismissive, or discouraging most of the time?
6. Do you plan ways to avoid them?
7. Do you feel a sense of relief when you are away from them?
8. Can you easily identify who those people are?
9. Why are they still in your life? What are your benefits from keeping them?

This exercise can help you become aware of some of the toxic people you might have in your life. Whether they are family member, co-workers, friends, or bosses, these people create a lot of discomfort and stress in your life. Becoming aware and identifying them can help you start an action plan or an exit strategy.

Any type of toxicity has a negative impact on your state of health. People around you should be encouraging, understanding, compassionate, and happy to hear good news. Just as your inner toxicity has a negative effect on you, so does the outer toxicity that comes from people around you. As Churchill said, "A pessimist sees the difficulty in every opportunity, while an optimist sees the opportunity in every difficulty."

Any relationship begins with us. When our lives are filled with positive feelings, we open our doors to honest communication and a respectful relationship. But when our lives are filled with anger, stress, anxiety, and guilt, we have some left over for others as well. When we feel good about ourselves, we don't have the need to be overly critical because we don't feel threatened by others. But when we feel bad or depressed, there will be a spill-over into our relationships.

A more positive state of mind allows us to see other positions and express ourselves in a more caring way. These principals of separate realities suggests that no two people see life in the same way. This fact helps us become more tolerant of different points of views, less critical, and less judgmental because we are less attached to considering only our own point of view. Once we understand that it is futile to attempt to change someone else's view, we will release many of the pressures that our relationships might experience.

This does not mean that we give up our beliefs, but rather we understand that our beliefs are derived from our own thought process, and if our information is different, then our conclusions would be different as well. So, "Let's agree to disagree." By listening without judgment, the other person will sense our respect for what they say, resulting in increased understanding and collaboration.

Meaningful relationships require conscious effort. Each relationship is like a bank account, meaning the more you put in, the stronger the relationship. Keeping promises and being supportive, positive, encouraging, and a good listener while taking time for the other person are just a few ways to make deposits. By keeping our emotional bank accounts growing, our relationship will be more meaningful and self-fulfilling.

Our relationships are mirrors of ourselves. What we attract are the qualities that we have. The things we don't like about people are the exact things that we don't accept within ourselves. We would not have those people in our lives if the way they are didn't somehow complement our own lives. For example, if you have a friend who lets you down and is undependable, looking closely at your life, you might find that in some areas you exhibit the same or similar traits.

When faced with a conflict, we need to ask ourselves, "What is this situation telling me about my own nature?" More often than not, the traits that bother us the most in another person are the ones we try hardest to deny in ourselves. As we embrace our darker qualities, we might be less inclined to judge someone else for expressing theirs. As we relinquish our judgment, we might see qualities that may be attractive in the other person that we have not allowed ourselves to see.

<u>Types of Relationships</u>

What type of people do you surround myself with: liberators who reinforce your growth or limiters who hinder it?

Liberators are people who support your desires for positive change by feeding you courage and confidence. Limiters are people who discourage you from taking life-expanding risks.

There are many different types of limiters who can hinder our progress in life. One is the **bully** who enjoys hurting us and looking good while making us feel bad. What lies beneath a bully is a poor self-image; while he is putting us down, the bully feels better about himself. They are weak, easily threatened, and cannot tolerate being ignored. Try to avoid them since they are toxic both to themselves and everyone around them.

The constant talker is another type of limiter. He never shuts up; he is argumentative and loud. Even when we try to say something, he will interrupt without listening to us. Constant talkers have no interest in whatever we have to say. It's hard to be around them because they never hear what we say. It's like hitting a brick wall. The constant talker knows it all can never go wrong and must have the last word. At times, they even lie to keep face. These people are relentless, so it's difficult to be around them as well.

The temper tantrum type is another type of limiter that screams, carries on, and slams the phone on us . They act like five-year-olds throwing temper tantrums. But remember that their outbursts are irrational and their apologies are meaningless. There's also the two-faced liar who spreads gossip and at times even makes up lies about us to look good. They are mean spirited, causing trouble among friends. They can easily stab us in the back, and they will say anything other than the truth.

How do we diffuse limiters' language? First we must recognize how their language affects us and make sure that the voice is not coming internally from within us. If we can eliminate them from our life, that's good, but if we cannot or we don't want to give them up, then we need to recognize their language and set limits to their negativity or confront their toxicity. We can defend ourselves with phrases such as, "I appreciate your feedback. Let me get back to you when I've had same time to think about it."

The same rules apply to our family members as well. Who is on board with us and who isn't? We need to recognize that some family members are going to be supportive of our changes, while others are not on the same page with us. We need to take a close look to see if our family members have achieved a certain psychological security about our decision to make changes in our life. If some feel insecure, then instead of being supportive, they might discourage us from making any changes. Remember that all the changes that we are about to make in our life will have a big impact on everyone else around us. So we might find out that not everyone is ready to participate in our process of change.

Exercise III

Signs to ditch a friend:

1. Is your friend draining you?
2. Is your friend judgmental, critical, and discouraging most of the time?
3. Is your friend dishonest?
4. Does your friend betray you?
5. Are you comfortable with yourself in the relationship?

These are a few simple questions that will help you get started. If your answers are "yes" to most of these questions, then it's time to be honest about the people that you keep around and ask yourself: Why are they still in my life? Remember, you are losing your core value in these relationships. It's time to move away, so move on with your life to seek out friends that you feel comfortable being around.

Keep your distance by maintaining your boundaries. Stay focused on your goals. Don't stoop down to their level of thinking or being. For example, if they come to you to unload about another friend, don't join in. Rather refocus the conversation by responding with more positive statements. Stand up for yourself, and don't feel obligated to remain close. Know what you want, and don't hesitate to ask for it. If you don't want to gossip, just say, "I am not interested in talking about Ruth when she is not present."

Having good authentic friends in our lives is important at any age, but especially in middle age. An authentic friend is understanding, encouraging, supportive, rewarding, easy, listens well, is accountable, and someone we can create real boundaries with. These are the types of friendship where we can lose touch for months and reconnect where we left off. With these type of friends, there is an upbeat quality that we all yearn for. When opportunity comes our way, we need to cherish it because being able to share our lives with another person who is a real friend is both liberating and comforting.

Rightsizing Your Finances

Will Rogers expressed our relationship with money eloquently: "Too many people spend money they haven't earned to buy things they don't want to impress people they don't like. (109)" Our relationship with money was developed early in our childhood years by watching those close to us deal with money. We have internalized those early messages and many of them became our present style of handling money. We use them without asking ourselves if they serve us well or they are self-defeating. What kinds of behaviors did we see around money? Did we see overspending, thriftiness, complete denial of spending habits, or financial enablers? Our first step is to understand our relationship with money and its origin to see if it's not self-defeating. Becoming aware of our earliest memories about money and examining our present relationship helps us make any necessary changes.

Exercise IV

Ask yourself:

What is my relationship with money?

What do I tell myself about money?

What type of spender am I?

What would I like to change in my own money mind-set? Why?

These few questions help you get in touch with your own money mind-set as well as the role money plays in your life. Does it serve you well or is it counter-productive. Do you stress over money? Does money worry you? Does it hinder your quality of life? Remember, a healthy relationship with money will set you free to earn, spend, save, and invest as you see fit.

Having a healthy relationship with money requires finding a balance between our rational and emotional mind-sets. This balance will give us the ability to judge for ourselves how much money we have at any given time and spend it wisely. A self-defeating mind set, such as "Money will give my life meaning" comes from a place of feeling deprived in our childhood years. As a result, we feel that money will give us respect. Our self-esteem is wrapped up with our bank accounts and salaries. On the one hand, feeling guilty about spending money on ourselves reflects our fear that we don't earn enough money and we don't deserve to take care of ourselves. Being an over-spender reflects our feelings of insecurity, or masks some of our inner chaos, such as stress, depression, loneliness, or helplessness. A healthy relationship with money will set us free from some of our inner chaos and give us more confidence in our ability to handle money well.

In her book *Three Guineas*, Virginia Woolf pointed to the importance of financial security without directly referring to it. She said that financial dependence and inexperience with money matters makes it harder for us to fully participate in the world. She called "having a room of our own" necessary for our self-fulfillment, which simply means that the formula for self-fulfillment was having money and a room of our own. Money and our ability to handle it is liberating on all levels.

We need to become familiar with our income, the requirements of our budgets, and the allocation of our money. Money management is an important skill that we all need to acquire to feel financially secure and in control of our lives.

Rightsizing Your Work Ethic

In a world that values the primacy of work, the most common question that we ask and get asked is what we do. Work enables us to express our talents, creativity, freedom as well as become self-sufficient. Making a decision about work is often a challenging one at middle age. But we all share one thing in common: work is where we find satisfaction, freedom, financial security, connections, and personal growth. Each one of us is trying to understand where our work fits in with our new discoveries about who we are at this stage of our lives.

As we consider different work options, such as early retirement, part-time work, changes in our careers or staying on the job full time, we need to realize that we are not the workers we were only older. Our outdated assumptions about what we expect and need from the work we do, as well as what we are prepared to bring to it, need to be updated. Our workplace has changed dramatically throughout the years. With all the modern technologies at our disposal, we need to adjust to those changes if we are to succeed. What's important at this stage of our lives is a job that caters to what matters to us now, including our needs, interests, work environment, and lifestyle. By middle age, we feel more comfortable in our ability to harmonize our public and private values and to combine our long-term and short-term goals, including work.

As we start reshuffling our priorities, work gains more flexibility. We can reduce our work hours to make room for the rest of our lives. We can change careers. We can start a new business. We can become more resourceful and sophisticated by using our acquired life experiences. We are better at recognizing our strengths and weaknesses and using them to our advantage. We can make changes in our lives and still stay connected to our skills and a steady paycheck. In my case, I love my job as a college professor, but doing it part time allows me to concentrate on other areas of my life, including family, hobbies, writing this book, and cultivating my friendships. It allows me to recalibrate my time, money, and life satisfaction, bringing harmony into my life.

De-Cluttering Your Time

To manage our time effectively means facing up to our cultural addiction to busyness, rushing, running, and multi-tasking. Actually, we take pride in our ability to multi-task better than men. We are all familiar with the saying, "Men are good at doing one thing at the time, while women can handle many tasks at the same time." But we pay a heavy price for this ability. It takes a toll on us both physically and mentally. We are taking on more responsibilities in less time, causing us stress, tiredness, anger, depression, sleep deprivation, and a general feeling of being run down. We run through life without taking a breath to enjoy it.

All these emanate from our cultural message that emphasizes productivity, work, possessions, and being useful. The first question we ask anyone we meet is what they do. This information gives us a rough estimate of how useful they are and how much money they make. But if we address the clutter in our minds, we realize that our continuous racing robs us of energy as well as mental and physical calmness. Earlier in this book I emphasized the importance of eliminating our stresses through mental calmness, exercise, meditation, good nutrition, and allowing our minds to do less and slow down. So being able to manage our time effectively and eliminating some of our stresses is important for both our mental and physical health.

If we examine closely what time is, we realize that it's nothing more than a mental construct. It's completely relative, and it's the result of our present focus. For example, how long is a long time? It depends on the situation. Sitting in traffic for one hour can seem like an eternity, while one hour with friends can pass quickly. Or when we become engrossed in something we enjoy, we lose track of time because we are no longer focused upon it. Now we are focused on something we like. What all this means is that we are in full control of our time, and by learning how to better allocate it we will make our lives easier and calmer. It's within our control to decide what to do with our time, and therefore with our level of personal fulfillment.

CHAPTER X

Your Anim-Morphosis from Goals to Actions

"By failure to prepare, you are preparing to fail".
Benjamin Franklyn

"Twenty years from now, you will be more disappointed by the things that you didn't do than by the ones you did."
Mark Twain

You have come a long way from where you were before you started reading this book. You have acquired valuable skills and knowledge on how to honestly look at yourself, your lifestyle, and your environment. You know that you are in charge of your thinking, feelings, and actions. If you have relinquished this power, it's time to reclaim it and start acting in your own best interest. Middle age is the perfect time to take a big plunge into the unknown and create a positive momentum for change, growth, and vitality.

It's time to move from awareness to action, from planning to acting. You have lived half of your life wishing, goal setting, and procrastinating. It's time to take control of your life and start living. It's time to get to work, discover your true self, your strengths, your weaknesses, your likes and dislikes, your dreams, your aspirations, and your joy. Getting real with yourself is the foundation for your existence. To have a different life, you need to do different, be different and think different. Your commitment to act will help you get the life that you want, since by now you know that the same old actions and thoughts will give you the same old results.

As the great poet Goethe said, "Whatever you can do or dream, you can begin it." This is your time to begin it. Set your course of action, and move from dreaming to actually doing. Remember, a strong you depends as much on what you do as on your ideas of yourself. For example, you can silence your inner critic, but if you feel helpless in the face of your dreams and need to change, then you may never fully accept yourself. A strong sense of self depends on learning to think in a healthy way and on your ability to make things happen and create what you want for yourself. Feeling helpless makes you angry, frustrated, and confused with your life. Only goal-oriented changes put you in charge of your life and destiny. So, ask yourself: what do I want? Once you know, find a way to achieve it.

If we think of our early adulthood as the years we built our lives, set our goals, formed our habits, beliefs, and lifestyle, we can think of middle age as our time to re-examine, re-evaluate, re-adjust, and challenge some of our decisions that might not work as well today as they did in the past. We need to find out whether those early decisions serve us well or hinder our lives. Since we are more experienced and wiser, we can easily recognize the things that don't work well in our lives and start fixing them.

Saying no to things that don't work is the assertive form of letting go and moving on. But there is a catch. The changes that we are about to make cannot be anticipated from the safety of our solid ground. We need to take risks and step into the unknown. We have to take the plunge into our middle age without a safety net, not knowing who we will become when we come up for air. I did it. It was exciting, challenging, and at times scary, but it was worth the risk.

This book is not about wanting or wishing for something, but rather it's geared toward challenging us to act. It's geared toward getting us out of the messes we created for ourselves and learning to take charge of our lives. Taking responsibility for our own destiny without any excuses will help us achieve a sense of empowerment and control over our lives. This type of rewarding action requires that we take risks by stepping outside our comfort zone and putting to the test our natural desire to feel secure. The rewards will be life-sustaining and invigorating. This is our time to get real about our lives and everyone in them.

We are all guilty of lying to ourselves about ourselves and our lives from time to time. Facing up to those lies will set us free. We all know how liberating it feels when we come clean and tell the truth. Living with a lie means we are distorting the truth about ourselves and we live in a state of complete denial. We can never get where we want to go until we acknowledge how dishonest we have been to ourselves and how we hinder our growth by looking in the wrong places for our answers. By looking head-on at our lives we will be able to shed the burden that is holding us back from realizing our dreams. No matter what's going on in our lives right now, our lives can be fixed if we are willing to fix them.

We start from the beginning with our thoughts. What are we telling ourselves? Are we being encouraging, supportive like a good parent would be, or are we being discouraging and critical? If our internal dialogue says, "I cannot do this. It's too late in my life," we are setting ourselves up for inaction. If we spend too much time focusing on the negatives, we feed our fears and starve our motivation. We end up stuck. Rather than fixating on why we can't, won't, or shouldn't do something, we need to continually remind ourselves why we can, will, and should pursue our dreams. Nothing is standing between you and your dreams except you.

Every day we are faced with different impediments. They are the goal stoppers that work on us 24/7. We use them to keep ourselves safe from the pain failing would cause us. This is an example of all-or-nothing thinking, which classifies us as either good at something or a complete failure. We don't feel comfortable with the middle ground. This type of thinking stops us from moving on because we need to be at the top. If not, we find it anxiety provoking, and we give up.

Another impediment could be choosing a goal to enrich our sense of validation by making us feel, sound, and look smarter. The danger with this type of thinking is that if we fail we believe that we don't have what it takes and give up. Refocusing our attention from being good to getting better and learning how to use our failure as feedback on how to improve (instead of devaluing ourselves) is our strongest motivator.

If we examine the difference between being good, which is tied to our self-worth, and getting better, which is tied to our self-improvement, we realize that becoming the most capable person is a much stronger and challenging motivational factor than just being good. The getting better goals are all about the journey to get there and accomplish what we set out to accomplish.

By focusing on growth instead of validation, on making progress instead of proving ourselves, we get further in life. D Bloom (1967) called these types of people "mastery oriented." They are able to handle setbacks since those setbacks don't represent their self-worth. They value learning. They are not afraid to fail, and failure does not threaten their sense of competence. They set up challenging goals, take risks, and they attribute success to their own efforts and abilities. They take credit for their success, and they accept their failure.

On the other hand, failure-accepting people think that their problems are due to their low ability and incompetence. They become helpless and give up. In the middle we have the failure-avoiding people who are afraid to fail, and their failure represents their self-worth. They use all types of excuses for their inaction. They are consumed by fear of failing, and they don't even try.

Goals also have to include the right balance between why we want to do something as well as what we need to do to accomplish it. Many of us set goals that seem good at the time, but become more and more awful as time goes by. For example, you agree to take your friend to the airport the same evening that you have a late presentation at work. Why is this happening to you more frequently than not? It's because when you set up your goal, you did not think much about whether or not you could pull it off. You did not take your time to consider what needs to be done and allocate your time appropriately. You might have concentrated more on why you want to take your friend to the airport instead of actually what you need to do to accomplish both goals.

If we adopt goals based on our motivation (such as our friend liking us) and not on what we have to do to accomplish it, we set ourselves up to fail. When we consider what we need to do, our goal becomes more realistic because we consider the time and the specific steps needed to accomplish it.

If we think of the why we want to do something, we start with an abstract kind of thinking because we are linking a particular action to a greater meaning or purpose. For example, saying that you will spend an extra hour at work three times a week to finish paperwork means that you are thinking of helping your career. You will be more motivated to stay longer on your job because you have a greater purpose.

When we think about what we are doing in why terms, we are guided by a bigger picture than our smaller actions, and our goal becomes part of something larger and more important. The why will energize and motivate us, while the what will get us focused on the exact steps needed to complete our task.

Goals that have intrinsic motivation, goals driven by our strong internal desires, are the once that are successful. These are the goals we want to accomplish regardless of any outside influences or pressures. Being free is our strongest motivator toward success because it satisfies our own need for autonomy and independence and reinforces our self-esteem. Any time we allow someone else to determine our sense of worth we give them permission to control our life. All intrinsically motivated goals will prove to be more powerful and longer lasting than externally driven ones. For example, we will be more likely to succeed in losing weight if we do it because we want to become healthier than if we are doing it to please our spouse.

Goal completion is also influenced by our self-acceptance and positive affirmation. Our positive attitude toward ourselves is a prerequisites for our goal accomplishments. Whenever those disruptive negative thoughts come into our minds we need to let them go by saying: "I approve of myself, and I accept myself." This phrase, if it's repeated many times each day, is a guaranteed way to bring up everything buried in our consciousness that is in opposition. Remember, our thoughts have no power over us unless we give in to them. So planting new seeds into our minds with strong positive affirmations will set us free from all the negativities that we have tolerated most of our lives.

By changing our minds, we are changing our lives. Whenever we get stuck on the way, we need to examine the reasons for being stuck. Is it because we live in the past moment? If we live in the past, many things could hold us back, such as fear, guilt, shame, stress, or anger. We need to remember that all those states of mind come from a place of refusal to let go and forgive ourselves and begin living in the present. Self-forgiveness and self-acceptance are always the answers to healing of any sort.

For any meaningful and sustainable changes, we need to ask ourselves what we want our lives to look like over the next few years and come up with a vision for our future. This vision will become our starting point for our planning. We make a lot of statements, but we don't follow them through. We all talk about the importance of maintaining our health as we age, but how many of us act on it? Or we talk about making changes in our lives, but how many of us follow through? We are good at making plans, but lousy at following them through. Planning is about what we will do. It begins with making a distinction between what can be changed versus what cannot be changed and then implementing it with our actions.

Create an Action Plan

How do we translate our plans into actions? Planning to do something only works if it's followed by action. We may want the results that the change will bring, but many of us are nowhere near ready to take action. Readiness is a way of assessing our willingness, desire, time, and energy to bring about that change. A good predictor of success is our self-efficacy, which is confidence that we have in our ability to succeed. For success we need to have a specific plan of action with clearly defined steps, as well as an ability to self-manage our thoughts, time, and action. We are more likely to try something new if we believe in ourselves and in our ability to succeed. The more we do, the more confidence we develop. Our readiness to change is really about weighing the desire to change against our resistance to change. Changing our old habits is hard. It takes hard work, time, and persistence.

There is no strategy more effective for fighting off saboteurs than doing a little advance planning. But not all plans work well for the simple reason that not enough thought goes into them. As the famous John Lennon said, "Life is what happens to you while you're busy making other plans." There is a good reason why some plans don't work.

Many times what we call a plan is nothing more than a laundry list. Let's take an example such as losing weight. A plan to lose weight would entail eating less and working out more. If we plan this way, it feels like we are making a plan, but in actuality all we are doing is listing the actions that we need to take in a general way. We have left out all the important details. When will we work out more? Where and how are we going to work out? What are we going to eat less of? How much less? What are we going to eat more of? Is this a good time to start my weight loss? Setting goals has a powerful impact on us if they are well thought out with specific details as to what, when, where and how to achieve them.

Setting up a specific plan of action and shifting our thinking from planning to creating a detailed strategy of action is the only way to achieve our goals. We don't reach goals by wishing for them. We make our dreams come true by creating a strategic plan of action and following it until we reach our desired goal. The moment we start taking our first steps, we might notice some of our fear promoters start working in our head. Phrases such as "need to," "should never," or "could never" start popping up. But you need to remember that the only person who thinks you should or should not do something is you.

To fight our blocking factors, we need to create a fearless thought for every fearful thought. "I should wait until my kids are older to start a new career" could be countered with "But if I do it now, I will have a better chance to get my dream job, and I will be in a better position to be involved with the kids when they are teens." Our fear responses are the oldest and strongest defenses that we use to protect ourselves from any type of discomfort. We need to be vigilant and catch them the minute they occur, stopping them with counter-sabotaging statements. Once we become more accustomed to our new ways of doing things, our fear responses will lose their power over us.

From Planning to Acting

Exercise I

Before you start your action, pause for a few minutes and ask yourself some important questions.

- Is this goal important right now?
- Am I ready to change?
- Do I want to devote time and energy to achieve it?
- Do I have access to the necessary resources to achieve it?
- Do I feel motivated enough at this time to actually achieve it?

If your answers are yes to all of these questions, then you are ready to proceed to the next step.

Create a specific action plan with step by step descriptions of what you need to do. When would you start? How much time do you need to accomplish it? What would it take for you, to reach your goal?

Monitor your progress. Make sure that you proceed on the right path. You are the only person that knows exactly what your goal involves. If you derail, you can get yourself back on the right track.

We all encounter bumps on our way. We need to give ourselves time for our success to take root. Patience and time will pay off in the long run. Let's not become discouraged by setbacks but rather use them as a learning tool. One failure is one failure, so let's stop globalizing. If you're bad at one thing, it doesn't mean you're bad at everything. Having setbacks is normal. The only difference is how we handle our failures and how we use our failure to define ourselves. Instead of thinking to yourself, "I'm a loser," next time you have a setback try telling yourself, "I did everything I could do, and next time around I will proceed differently. It's a good lesson for the future." This type of self-compassion helps us eliminate anger, fear, depression, guilt, shame, and the pain we might experience when things go wrong. Being able to accept responsibility for a negative event and not internalize it with a lot of negativity is important to keeping us going. We need to see ourselves kindly regardless of whether our goal turns out well or not.

Success is a series of trials and errors. If at first we don't succeed, try again. All this means that instead of beating ourselves up for our errors, we should be more focused on learning from them and trying another way until we get it right. If we settle for mediocrity, we are not using our full potential to reach our dreams. We are operating with an empty tank, selling ourselves short by settling for less than what we can actually achieve. Let's start acting and taking charge of our lives.

Achieving isn't just about being able to reach our goal but also the pursuit of our goals to reach our fullest potential in life. As Carl Rogers said, most of us don't reach our full potential, and we are operating with a half-empty tank. We miss the thrill that the process of getting there gives us. Our belief in our ability as well as our progress in achieving our dreams is a strong motivator. If we believe that ability is a quality that we can develop through learning and experience, then we can succeed. But if we live under the false assumption that our abilities are fixed and, no matter what we do, we will not improve, we are closed to the concept of improving. Embracing the accurate belief that we can change even our ability will allow us to make good choices.

Improve Your Self-Management Skills

Exercise II

- Change your mind-set; small success is better than no success.
- Change your inner dialogue.
- Develop positive affirmations to counter your fears, anxieties, and uncertainties.
- Replace fear-motivated behavior with acceptance. Fear is a product of your past. Live in the present to create your future.
- Break your addictions that paralyze you. Every type of dependency slows you down and dulls your life.
- Recognize your excuses.
- Don't be afraid to fail. Failure is a part of your learning curve.
- Start creating your best life possible. Any changes in your life require your action, not your wishing or dreaming.
- Live in the present, and become mindful of your thinking, feeling, and action.

Today you are equipped with more information, knowledge, understanding, experience, and self-awareness than ever before. You have moved successfully from ignorance in infancy to wisdom in middle adulthood. You fully understand the strong interconnection that exists between your body and mind. You understand that you cannot flourish physically if you are weak mentally, or vice versa. You have developed a strong sense of self-awareness, self-acceptance, and self-love which are the basic foundations for your personality. You have learned how to disarm and silence you inner critical voice that kept discouraging you from realizing your dreams.

You cultivated flexibility and creativity by maintaining a healthy body and mind. You have learned how to stop your biological clock by taking care of your body and mind with physical exercise, proper nutrition, and mental activity. You have acquired knowledge on healthy foods. You have learned that the food that you eat every day has an enormous impact on your health and could keep you disease free. Nurturing your body and mind with healthy foods and exercise is the best anti-aging medication on the market today, and it's free for you to use.

You have learned that nurturing your body from the outside with self-grooming and self-care improves both your physical and mental health. You know that if you take care of your inner self, it will reflect on your outside appearance, and vice versa. If you feel good about yourself, it will reflect on your body, face, hair, clothing, and your general self-grooming.

You understand the importance of keeping harmony in your life by eliminating all sources of toxicity. Too much clutter, toxicity, chaos, and dissonance in your life creates a stressful, unhealthy environment that hinders your existence. You have learned how to bring balance and calm into your life by rightsizing your life, by cleaning your house internally as well as externally.

235

But the most important lesson that you have learned is knowing how to implement all these skills and put them into action. How you accomplish it all is your choice since you are writing your own script. The second most important lesson that you have learned by reading this book is trusting yourself and your inner power to accomplish it all. You have confidence in your ability, and you are ready to create your own life list. So start working.

Conclusion

"We are what we repeatedly do."

Aristotle

"Anyone who has experienced something is more expert in it than the experts."

Gloria Steinem

"I am what survives me."

Erick Erikson

Imagine if you could gather the greatest minds in the field of anti-aging and learn what they themselves do to ensure that they live the longest and the healthiest lives possible. If you could find out what they do, what they eat, how they handle their stress, conflicts, challenges, and changes, you could adopt those strategies. Some of this important information is gathered in this book for your use.

This book equips you with important information on how to navigate through middle age and beyond. It clarifies some of the confusions, contradictions, misinformation, and misleading negative messages that society directs at middle-aged women—messages that hinder your quality of life. It clarifies the numerous natural changes that you experience throughout your aging process. It clarifies the negativities and dissatisfactions that you might encounter at this point of your life, as well as clearly defines middle age and its different sub-stages.

If there is a specific time that we call middle age, then what is it? When does it start and when does it end? Do we all go through it at the same time and have similar experiences? What distinguishes some of us who look fifty from others who look seventy with the same chronological age? What distinguishes those of us who sustain our stamina and youthful looks from those that do not? How can we navigate through own aging process without any clear understanding of its onset, duration, and progression? How can we go through life without a clear understanding of this long life span called middle age? And why is so little attention paid to its developmental course? It starts in our late forties and it extends into our early seventies. All these questions and many more are addressed throughout this book, giving you a clear understanding of your aging process.

Just as our adolescence connects our childhood years with our early adulthood, middle age connects our early adulthood with our old age. Middle age is a significant life span with many distinct and visible changes similar to the ones we experienced during our adolescent years. Both in middle age and adolescence we see visible changes on our faces, bodies, energy level, behaviors, emotions, feelings, and attitudes. If we attribute all these visible changes to getting old, then we take no responsibility for our unfolding lives, and we accept everything that comes our way as a natural progression of things to come. We tell ourselves this is the way things are; we're just getting old.

More and more of us benefit from the vast body of information available on better nutrition, physical and mental activity, de-stressing, better sleep, and regular physical checkups, but not everyone. Others are stuck believing that age is the only problem with their unhappy existence. They are locked into inaction with unhealthy nutrition, unhealthy lifestyles, unhealthy thinking, unhealthy habits, stress, distorted feelings, irrational beliefs, and unhealthy behaviors. They let their lives unfold without taking any responsibility for it.

This is the time to ask ourselves: do we want to educate ourselves and learn everything available to us, or stay stuck? If our answer is the former, then the rest will follow. This book emphasizes this simple reality and guides us toward acquiring this type of self-awareness and improving our quality of life. This is the time to do something or lag behind in the darkness without taking any responsibility for our lives.

The basic philosophy adopted throughout this book is anchored on the strong inter-connection that exists between you, the change you're making, and your aging process. You need all three components to function well in order to live the longest and healthiest life possible. You need a healthy sense of self-awareness, self-acceptance, and self-understanding, as well as constant growth. It all starts with you and your inner wellbeing since you create your entire life's script.

Age is not your enemy. Age can be used to work for you if you become well-informed of all the possibilities available to you. You can live well at any age. Since you are in charge, you decide what you want or don't want to change at any time.

I became interested in winning the aging process when I got into my late forties and early fifties. Through my research and experience as a psychologist and professor of psychology over many years, I acquired a deep understanding of aging and our lifecycles. This book is the product of those pursuits, providing you with guidance and ground-breaking knowledge on how to maintain a healthy and productive lifestyle at any age. I like to think of myself as a work in progress, with two feet moving forward and one moving backward. But with each new step that I take, I am convinced that I want this process of anim-morphosis to continue throughout my entire lifespan.

All this does not mean that I want to minimize our natural aging process, our gray and thinning hair, our wrinkles, the aches and pains caused by wear and tear in our bodies, but rather I argue that by extending our knowledge of our aging process and learning new ways to compensate for the inevitable changes that our aging brings, we can reverse our process of aging and sustain a healthier life into our late middle age.

Getting older every year is a given, but symptoms of aging are optional. It's empowering to know that how we age is determined by how we live, think, act, and feel. Since our genes control only one part of our aging process, the rest is up to us. Knowledge about our own aging process is the greatest present we can give ourselves at middle age to fight both our inner doubts and our cultural undertow that continues to regard our fifties as an inevitable decline.

Our society looks upon beauty and strength as qualities that we possess in our twenties and thirties while life beyond that is a downhill process. Our life is portrayed as a slow loss of vitality, creativity, curiosity and health. But let's not be drawn into these warped societal messages. Let's not become helpless but rather empower ourselves by focusing on the roots of our problems, which most of the time are things that we can control as opposed to aging, which we cannot.

Our society feeds us a lot of negativity about aging and in particular middle age. We buy into it and develop distorted beliefs about our own aging process that keep us stuck and unhappy. We look at ourselves as old, which soon becomes an easy explanation for many of our problems, and we give up. So when we feel aches and pain, gain weight, feel tired, or have low energy we attributed it all to getting old. We begin to accept it, live accordingly, and soon it becomes our self-fulfilling prophecy.

This book challenges all the negativity directed at aging and looks at the process of aging as a natural, healthy progression of living well. So let's not buy into the negativity that our society has instilled in us, but rather celebrate every age as a gift of life and make every year the most informative year of our lives.

Our new learning, curiosity, and inquiring mind redefines our cultural understanding of middle age and beyond. This book brings to light the purposeful learning that goes on in our middle adulthood and recognizes that age is not our enemy but rather a continuation of our adult years. It's an important part of our lifecycle in which we continue to express curiosity about our lives and our changing world. As Erikson(1967) argued, life is a continuous process of development that does not stop until the day we die.

I strongly disagree with the saying, "As I am getting older, I am becoming wiser" because it's not always the case. Getting older is a matter of age, but getting wiser is a matter of individual choice. We can take charge of our lives, or we can take the easy way out, do nothing, and suffer the consequences as they occur. But our generation of women is paving the way for all future generations by demonstrating resilience, thirst for learning, and determination to fight off societal condemnation for being too impulsive if we admit our lust for new discoveries.

While some of us might agree that women our age should be integrating all that they have learned and accomplished and take it easy without engaging in risk-taking projects and new ventures with a childlike enthusiasm, others, myself included, are eager to continue learning, exploring new avenues, and discovering new unfamiliar territories. Our generation of women is challenging and changing cultural beliefs through our sense of what's appropriate and inappropriate about the normal trajectories of aging. These new realities are reflected in our new educational attainments, living longer, having better health care, developing improved diets, engaging in more activities, and taking advantage of new medical interventions.

It seems that in every century a new developmental phenomenon emerges. Last century we focused our attention on adolescent development while in the 21st century middle age has emerged as a distinct and significant new period in development. This is a period between our young adulthood and old age, and we are redefining and challenging our cultural definitions of strength, power, and maturity. We are the baby boom generation, and we are making a noticeable impact on our society by challenging the definition of middle age and its appropriateness at every level possible. We are putting middle-age youthfulness on the map.

Documentaries and research offer inspiring narratives of our generation's carving out of new careers, having renewed confidence, and taking on new challenges in searching for greater meaning in life. Our culture still struggles with where exactly to place us, but our strong determination to learn reflects our strong response to our culture's ambivalence. Our generation is reshaping our cultural understanding of learning, stamina, wisdom, and productivity. We are actively engaged in the world around us, seeking out new opportunities for continued growth.

The fascinating aspect of middle age is that we can look back and move forward. For me, moving forward means crossing borders into new territories, which means a new way of thinking and acting. It forces me to learn new skills, try on new personas, and reinvent myself many times over. Moving forward fills my life with curiosity to find new ways of being in the world. Soon I realized that my new life doesn't exclude my old self and I am able to find a way to embrace the new with the old and construct something whole as I progress through my new journey of anim-morphosis. Through my journey, I find that my path is moving me forward and circling back, progressing and regressing, being both constant and changing. At times, I experience a sense of uncertainty, but within myself I find a new sense of freedom and courage that helps me move on.

When I began to write this book, I thought of it as my personal journey through middle age. But as time progressed, I realized that this book is more than that. It is a valuable contribution to my generation of women who are struggling to make sense of their own aging process. You can think of age as a life-long experience, where the more you put in, the more you take out. It's about creating the life you want by shifting your youth-oriented focus and discovering the wisdom of your age. Remember that middle age is your longest life span. It starts in your late forties and it extends until your early seventies. So you can either look at it as a life event that you must endure, or it could become an opportunity for change and growth.

Epilogue

The great Greek philosopher Socrates said, "The unexamined life is not worth living." This book is based on the same philosophical principle, which I call anim-morphosis. Change is a prerequisite at every age. Without re-examining, rediscovering, challenging, and making the necessary changes throughout your lifecycle, you are denying your full potential toward a healthy and vigorous life. Once you stop growing and developing, you stop living and become merely a survivor.

This book is a comprehensive guide that addresses different topics, questions, issues, and confusions that women face at middle age and beyond. Even though I cannot predict what it will it be like for you at this stage of your life, since your future is in your hands and not mine, I truly hope that this book will provide you a guiding light and a source of inspiration, knowledge, information, ideas, and exercises at this important juncture of your life.

You will decide what aspects of this book you want to use, how to use it, and how much time and energy are you willing to put into it as well as how committed, focused, and motivated you will be throughout your work. The results will be a clear reflection of your determination to bring about those changes in your life. Remember, you alone are in charge of your wellbeing. If your life is spinning out of control, this is the time to take back the steering wheel and take charge of your life. Don't relinquish your inner power or allow others to dictate your life's destiny.

My purpose in writing this book is not to pretend that it's possible to quickly navigate through the turbulent years of middle age because the process of change is never an easy one. Nor is this book intended to oversimplify your aging process or suggest that if you do such and such you will be fine. Rather it's a profound source of information that guides you toward a more meaningful life. It offers optimistic, practical, and sometimes playful techniques on how to face up to societal challenges, confusions, contradictions, and progress through our life transitions with courage.

I can only tell you how I have benefited from the changes that I have made. I started by healing some of my past pain and focused on the present. I became less critical and angry. I learned to appreciate life and everything that I have. I make every day count. I became more self-aware and accepting of my assets as well as my limitations. I started to look at health as a gift of life. I learned to relax, appreciate myself, and take time for myself without feeling guilty. I have eliminated most of my toxicities and chaos. I became less needy, more independent, and I enjoy spending time in my own company. I like to spend quality time with my husband, children, and my six grandchildren. I work out five days a week, which energizes me both physically and mentally.

I also realize that writing this book has been the most self-nurturing thing that I could have done for myself. This book serves me as a catalyst toward a fuller and more rewarding life at middle age.

Now, ask yourself: "What would it be like for you if you became a true friend to yourself and took life into your own hands?"

It would depend on how motivated you are, how much energy you are willing to put into changing certain aspects of your life, and how much faith you have in yourself that you actually can bring about those changes. You are not responsible for what happened to you in the past, but you are responsible for what you do or don't do with your life today. Your strength, determination, courage, and willingness to change those things that hinder your life will be sufficient to make you an expert on your own life. Once you have accomplished it, you are on your way to living the life that you always dreamed for yourself.

Bibliography

Adler, Alfred._Understanding Human Nature. Oxford: One World, 1992.

_____ . Individual Psychology. New York: Harper Press, 1952.

Amen, Daniel. Use Your Brain to Change Your Age. New York: Three Rivers Press, 2012.

_____. Change Your Brain Change Your Body. New York: Harmony Books, 2008.

Bandura, Albert. Self-Efficacy: The Exercise of Control. New York: Freeman Press, 1969.

_____. The Social Foundation of Thought and Action. N.J: Prentice Hall, 1986.

Bankson, Marjory. Creative Aging: Rethink Retirement and Non-Retirement in A Changing World. Woodstock, VT:Skylight, 2010.

Barash Shapiro, Susan. Toxic Friends. New York: St. Martin's Press, 2009.

Bateson, Mary. Composing a Further Life. New York: Knopf, 2010.

Baumeister R. & Exlin, J. Self-Control Morality and Human Strength. "Journal of Social and Clinical Psychology, 19, 2000, pp.29-42.

Becklin, Linda. Come Rain Or Come Shine: Friendship Between Women. New York: Adams Media, 1999.

Begoun, Paula. The Original Beauty Bible. Renton, Washington: Beginning Press, 2009.

Bendheim, Paul. The Brain Training Revolution. Il: Source Books, 2009.

Benneth, W. *Beyond Overeating.* "New England Journal of Medicine," 332, 1995, pp.673-674.

Berne, Erick. *Games People Play: The Psychology of Human Relationships.* London: Penguin Books, 1964.

Blanchard, Fields. *Everyday Problem Solving and Emotions. in "* Current Directions in Psychological Science, 16, 2007, pp.26-31.

Brander, Nathaniel. *The Psychology of Self-Esteem.* New York: Wiley, 1969.

_____ . *Honoring the Self.* New York: Bantam Books, 1990.

Braverman, Eric. *Younger You: Unlock the Hidden Power of Your Brain to Look and Feel 15 Years Younger.* New York: McGraw Hills, 2007.

Bridges, Williams. *Making Sense of Life's Changes.* Reading, Mass: Addison-Wesley, 1980.

Brokan, Sara. *Fortytide: Making the Next Decades the Best Years of Your Life through the 40's, 50's and Beyond:* New York:Voice, 2011.

Brown, Lyn & Gilligan, Carol. *Meeting at the Crossroads: Women's Psychology and Girls Development.* Cambridge, Mass: Harvard University Press, 1992.

Burns, David. *Feeling Good: The New Mood Therapy.* William Morrow, 1980.

Cash, T. & Henry, P. *Women's Body Images.* "Journal of Sex- Roles," 33, 1995, pp.19-28.

Carper, Jean. *Stop Aging Now. The Ultimate Plan for Staying Young and Reversing the Aging Process.* New York: Harper Perennial, 1996.

Chittister, Joan. *The Gift of Years: Growing Older Gracefully.* New York: Bluebridge Books, 2008.

Chopra, Deepak. *Ageless Body Timeless Mind.* New York: Harmony Books, 1993.

_____-. *Unconditional Life.* New York: Bantam Books,1991.

_____. *Perfect Health: The Complete Mind Body Guide.* New York: Three Rivers Guide. 2000.

Cohen, Gene. *The Mature Mind: The Positive Power of the Aging Brain.* New York: Basic Books,2005.

Cohen, Patricia. *In Our Prime: The Invention of the Middle-Age.* New York: Scribner, 2012.

Coleman, D. *Working With Emotional Intelligence.* New York: Bantam Books,2010.

Cottin, Pogrebian. *Getting Over Getting Older.* Boston: Little Brown Co., 1996.

Csikszentmihaly, M. *Creativity Flow and the Psychology of Discovery.* New York: Harper Collins, 1996.

Deci, E. *Facilitating Optimal Motivation and Well-Being Across Life's Domain.* Canadian Psychology, 2008.

Deep, Sam. *What To Say To Get What You Want.* New York: Addison-Wesley, 1992.

Dement, W. *The Promise of Sleep.* New York: Delacorte Press, 1999.

Diener, E. *Beyond Money: Toward An Economy of Well-Being.* Psychological Science in the Public Interest, 2004.

Diller, Vivian. *Face It: What Women Really Feel as Their Looks Changes.* New York: Hay House, 2010.

Dixon, R. *Memory and Aging.* "Canadian Psychology," 48, 2007, pp. 67-76.

Dostoevsky, Fyodor. *Crime and Punishment, 1886.*

Down, Hugg. *Fifty Forever.* Nashville, Tenn: Thomas Nelson, 1994.

Dreker, H. *The Immune Power Personality.* New York: Dutton, 1995.

Drukman, D. *In the Minds' Eye: Enhancing Human Performance.* Washington, D.C: National Academic Press,, 1991.

Dychtward, Ken. *Age Power: How the 21ᵗʰ Century Will Be Ruled by the New Old.* New York: Jeremy Tracher, 2000.

Eagly, A. *Female Leadership: Advantages and Disadvantages.* "Psychology of Women's Quarterly, 31, 2007.

Edelman, Hope. *Motherless Daughters.* Boston: De Capo Press, 2006.

Einstein. G. *Normal Aging and Perspective Memory.* " Journal of Experimental Psychology," 16, 1995, pp. 717-726, 1995.

Ellis, Albert. *New Guide to Rational Living.* New York: Institute for Rational-Emotive Therapy, 1975.

Emmons, Robert. *The Psychology of Gratitude.* New York: Oxford University Press, 2004.

Ephron, Nora. *I Remember Nothing.* New York: Knopf, 2010.

Erdelyi, M. *Psychoanalysis: Freud's Cognitive Psychology.* New York: Freeman, 1985.

Erikson, Erik. *Childhood and Society.* New York: Norton, 1963.

_____. *Identity: Youth and Crisis.* New York: Norton, 1968.

_____. *Adulthood.* New York: Norton, 1978.

Erikson, Erik & Joan Erikson. *The Life Cycle Complete: Extended Version.* New York: Norton, 1998.

Erikson, Erik & Kivnick, Helen. *Vital Involvement in Old Age.* New York: Norton, 1986.

Fletcher, Kate. *Fashion and Sustainability: Design of Change.* London: Laurence King Publishers, 2012.

Fonda, Jane. *My Life So Far.* New York: Random House, 2005.

Foster, Stanley. *The Toxic Executive.* New York: Harper, 1993.

Forward, Susan. *Emotional Blackmail: When People in Your Life Use Fear and Guilt to Manipulate You.* New York: Harper Collins, 1996.

Freedman, Mask. *Prime Time: How Baby Boomers Will Revolutionize Retirement.* New York: Public Affairs, 2000.

_____. *Second Half of Life.* New York: Public Affairs, 2007.

Freud, Sigmund. *The Interpretation of Dreams.* Oxford: Oxford University Press, 1900.

_____. *Inhibitions Symptoms and Anxiety.* New York: Norton, 1959.

Friedan, Betty. *The Fountain of Age.* New York: Simon & Schuster, 1993.

_____. *The Feminine Mystique.* New York: Norton, 1997.

Gardner, Howard. *Frames of Mind: The Theory of Multiple Intelligence.* New York: Basic Books, 1983.

Gilbert, D. *Stumbling On Happiness.* New York: Knopf, 2006.

Gill, Libby. *You Unstuck.* Palo Alto, California: Solas House, 2003.

Gilligan, Carol. *In a Different Voice: Psychological Theory & Women's Development.* Cambridge, Mass: Harvard University Press, 1993.

_____. *The Birth of Pleasure.* New York: Knopf, 2002.

Glass, Lilian. *Toxic People.* New York: St. Martin's Press, 1995.

Gladwell, Malcolm. *Blink: The power of Thinking Without Thinking.* London: Penguin, 2005.

Goodman, Ellen. *I Know Just What You Mean: The Power of Friendship in Women's Lives.* New York: Simon &Schuster, 2002.

Goleman, Daniel. *Working With Emotional Intelligence.* London: Bloomsbury, 1998.

Gratzer, W. *Terrors on the Table: The Curious History of Nutrition.* Oxford: Oxford University Press, 2005.

Guiliano, Mineille. *French Women Don't Get Fat.* New York: Knopf, 2001.

Harlow, Harry. *The Nature of Love.* "American Psychologist," 13, 1958, pp.573-685.

Helson, Ravena. *Personality Change in Women from Early 40's to the Early 50's.* "Psychology of Aging," 7, 1992, pp. 193-203.

Hendles, S. *"The Complete Guide to Anti-Aging Nutrition.* New York: Simon & Schuster, 1984.

Hillman, J. *The Force of Character and the Lasting Life.* New York: Random House, 1996.

Hollis, James, *Finding Meaning in the Second Half of Life.* New York: Gotham Books, 2006.

_____. *The Middle-Passage: From Misery to Meaning in Midlife.* Toronto: Inner City Books, 1993.

Horney, Karen. *Our Inner Conflicts.* London: Routladge & Kegan, 1957.

_____. *Feminine Psychology.* New York: Norton, 1967.

Huitsch, D. *Use It Or Lose It.* "Psychology of Aging," 14, 2007, pp.245-263.

Irmside, Virginia. *Twenty Reasons Why Growing Old Is Great.* New York: A Plime Book, 2009.

James, Hollis. *The Middle Passage.* Toronto: Inner City Books, 1993.

James, William. *The Principle of Psychology.* New York: Dover,1950.

Jung, Carl. *Memories, Dreams, Reflections.* New York: Vintage Books, 1965.

Katch, W. *Essentials of Exercise Physiology.* Philadelphia, Wolters, 2011.

Kermis, M. *Toward the Conceptualization of Optimal Self-Esteem.* "Psychological Inquiry," 8, 2003, pp.2003.

Levine, Suzanne. *Inventing the Rest of Our Lives: Women in Second Adulthood.* New York: A Plumer Book, 1995.

Levy, B. *Longevity Increased by Positive Self-Perception of Aging.* "Journal of Personality and Social Psychology," 10, 2002, pp.261-270.

Locke, E. *The Theory of Goal Setting and Task Performance. N.J.: Prentice Hall, 1990.*

Maquet, P. *The Role of Sleep In Learning and Memory.* Science," 12, 2001, pp. 1048-52.

Marla, Paul. *The Friendship Crisis: Finding and Keeping Friends When You Are Not A Kid Anymore.* New York: Rodale, 2004.

Maslow, Abraham. *Toward a Psychology of Being.* Princeton, N.J: Van Nostrand, 1962.

Mehment, C. *You Staying Young.* New York: Free Press, 2007.

Miller, Baker. *Toward A New Psychology of Women. Boston: Beacon Press, 1976.*

Moreno, Mike. The 17 Day Plan to Stop Aging. New YorK; Free Press, 2012.

Nepo, Mark. *The Book of Awakening: Having the Life You Want By Being Present To the Life You Have.* Berkley, CA: Conari Press, 2000.

Neugarten, Berice. *Middle-Age And Aging.* Chicago: University of Chicago Press, 1968.

Nicolai, June. *Integrative Wellness Rules: A Simple Guide To Healthy Living.* CA: Hay House, 2013.

Northrop, Christine. *Mother-Daughter Wisdom.* New York: Bantam Books, 2005.

Oaten, Megan. *Improvement In Self-Control and Financial Monitoring.* "Journal of Economic Psychology," 12, 2007, pp. 68-80

Painter, Charlotte. *Gift of Age.* San Francisco: Chronicle's Books, 1985.

Peale, Norman. The Power of Positive Thinking. New York: Simon & Schuster,2003.

Pederson, Rena. What Next? Women Redefining Their Dreams in the Prime of Life. New York: Perigree Books, 2001.

Pearls, Fritz. *Gestalt Therapy: Excitement and Growth in the Human Personality.* London: Souvenir, 1951.

Piaget, Jean. *The Language and Thought of the Child.* London: Routlage & Kegan, 1959.

Pinker, S. *The Blank Slate: The Modern Denial of Human Nature.* London: Penguin, 2003.

Pinkola, Estes. *Women Who Run With the Wolves.* New York: Ballantine Books, 1992.

Planck, Nina. *Real Food: What To Eat and Why.* New York: Bloomsbury, 2006.

Polivy, J. *Psychological Consequences of Food Restrictions.* "Journal of American Diet," 96, 1996, pp. 589-592.

Pollan, Michael. *In Defense of Food.* New York: Penguin Books, 2009.

Raines, Howel. *Fly Fishing Through Midlife Crises.* New York: William Morrow, 1993.

Ratey, J. *The Revolutionary New Science of Exercise and the Brain.* New York: Little, Brown, 2008

Redford, Williams. *Anger Kills.* New York: Harper Torch, 1998.

Rentsch, Gail. *Smart Women Don't Retire—The Break Free.* New York: Springboard Press 2008.

Rodin, J. *Body Traps.* New York: William Morrow, 1992.

Roger, Carl. *ON becoming a PERSON: a Therapist View of Psychotherapy.* Boston: Houghton Mifflin, 1961.

Rubin, Lillian. *Uncharted Territory: Living the New Longevity.* Boston: Beacon Press, 2007.

Salmon, P. *Effects of Physical Exercise on Anxiety, Depression and Stress.* "Clinical Psychology Review, 15, 2001, pp. 36-61

Shapiro, Gail. *Money Order: The Money Management Guide for Women. New York: Simon & Schuster, 1975.*

Shapiro, Patricia. *Heart Deepening: Women's Friendships at Middle Life.* Berkeley CA: Berkeley Publishers, 2001.

Schwartz, Barry, *The Paradox of Choice: Why More Is Less.* New York: Harper Collins, 2004.

Seligman, Martin. *Learned Optimism.* New York: Knopf, 1999.

_____. *Authentic Happiness.* New York: Free Press, 2003.

Selye, Hans. *Stress Without Distress.* In G. Serban ed., "Psychopathology of Human Adaptation, New York: Plenum, 1976.

Sheely, Gail. *Passages.* New York: Bantam Books, 1974.

_____. *New Passages: Mapping Your Life Across Time.* New York: Random House, 1995.

Skinner, B. *Science and Human Behavior.* New York: MacMillan, 1953.

Snyder, C. & Lopez, S. *Positive Psychology: The Scientific and Practical Explanation of Human Strength.* CA: Sage, 2007.

Somer, Elizabeth. *Food and Mood: The Complete Guide to Eating Well and Feeling Your Best.* New York: A Holt Paperback, 1999.

Stanness, J. & Jenkins, M. *Eating Like A Woman and Never Diet Again.* New York: Harlequin, 2014.

Steinem, Gloria. *Revolution From Within: A Book of Self Esteem.* Boston: Little, Brown and Co., 1992.

Tanner, Deborah. *You Just Don't Understand: Women and Men in Conversations.* New York: Harper, 1990.

Trafford, A. *My Time: Making the Most of the Rest of Your Life.* New York: Basic Books, 2003.

Tribole, Evelyn. *Intuitive Eating: A Revolutionary Program that Works.* New York: St. Martin's Press, 2002.

Vailland, George. *Aging Well : Surprising Guide to a Happy Life.* Boston: Little, Brown, 2002.

Viscott, David. *Emotionally Free.* New York: Contemporary Books, 1993.

Vygotsky, L. *Mind In Society.* Cambridge, Mass: Harvard University Press, 1989.

_____. *Thought and Language.* Cambridge: The Mitt Press, 1989.

Wansink, Brian. *Mindless Eating: Why WE Eat More Than We Think.* New YorK Bantam Books, 2006.

Weil, Andrew. *Healthy Aging. A Lifelong Guide to Your Physical and Spiritual Wellbeing.* New York: Knopf, 2005.

Weinman, Martha. *Where Did I Leave My Glasses: The What, When and Why of Normal Memory Loss.* New York: Grand Central Pub. 2008.

Woolf, Virginia. *A Room of One's Own.* New York: Harcourt, Brace, 1929.

Wray, Herbert. *Outsmarting Your Mind: Hard Wired Habits.* New York: Crown Publishers, 2010.

Young, Erica. *Fear of Fifty: A Midlife Memoir.* New York: Harper Spotlight, 1995.

Index

About the Author

Dr. Lea Ausch Alteras holds a Ph.D. in Psychology from the City University of New York (CUNY) Graduate Center as well as a Psychoanalytic degree from the Psychoanalytical Institute of New York. She has been a Professor at Hunter College (CUNY) in New York teaching courses in Women's Studies, Educational Psychology as well as conducting research on Women's Aging Process in different cultures. She has been in private practice for many years specializing in women's periods of transitional development. In addition, Dr. Ausch is the author of a book, Three Generations of Jewish Women: Holocaust Survivors, Daughters and Granddaughters, as well as articles and reviews in scholarly journals in the United States and abroad. With the fall of communism she traveled in Eastern Europe conducting research as well as participated in conferences dealing with the changes in women's lives under the new social order. As the coordinator of Eastern European Women's Association in Hungary and Romania she was invited as guest speaker on issues relating to women's rights, such as abortion laws, child care, career training and education.

www.ingramcontent.com/pod-product-compliance
Lightning Source LLC
Chambersburg PA
CBHW030422290526
45786CB00001B/88